INTRODUCTUON

What Is Erectile Dysfunction?

If you are reading this book, chances are that you already know what erectile dysfunction is. To really get the most out of this book, I am going to briefly cover what ED actually is - simply so you can get a clear understanding and it will also speed up the entire process.

Erectile dysfunction is also known as male impotence and it happens in men, regardless of age. It is an issue wherein a male is unable to create or maintain an erection to perform sexual intercourse. A lot of people have first hand experience of it at some point. But what about that popular guy who dated that model in high school? Yep, he definitely had his struggles with ED too at some point in the bedroom.

So, don't take it personally, drop the victim mentality and don't think you're less of a man. There's more to being a man than maintaining an erection. And now that I've made my point, for the rest of the book we're going to focus on getting those rock-solid erections again. Erectile dysfunction is not part of aging because there are younger males who also suffer from it (although age is a risk factor). It can be an embarrassing condition but there are lots of ways to go about solving this issue.

There are men who presently suffer temporary impotence which is due to a lot of things. Depending on its cause, this however lasts only for an hour to just a few weeks. When you are extremely mentally or physically exhausted, you can suffer temporary impotence. Another cause is being exposed to hot or cold temperatures. If your genitalia have suffered injury like blunt trauma or you have undergone pelvic or spinal surgery, temporary erectile dysfunction may happen.

There are times when erectile dysfunction is a result of another health condition which you do not know you are suffering. In order to diagnose ED, you need to undergo a physical exam. Your doctor will note down all your symptoms and then evaluate them. He may also extract from you a blood sample so that he can check your levels of male hormones.

He may also ask you to undergo an ultrasonography to see if blood flows to your penis. He will also perform a cavernosometry so as to examine your penis' vascular pressure. You may also be asked to undergo neurologic evaluations to see if there if your genital nerves have suffered any injury or damage.

In a later chapter, I will offer you a simple test to determine whether your erectile dysfunction is a physical or mental issue.

Erectile dysfunction can be induced by many different causes. As previously mentioned, it may be caused by an underlying health condition, a mental or emotional problem (including relationship troubles), a side effect from current medications, a result of bad habits such as smoking, taking drugs, and drinking too much alcohol, or a combination of any of them. Constricting of the penile artery that prevents erection is most often caused by diabetes or can be a sign of a coronary artery condition as well. If this is the case, then receiving proper diagnosis and treatment of the principal cause should be the main priority.

Some prescription drugs and medicines could also cause erectile dysfunction. If there are any indications that your inability to hold an erection is caused by your current medications, then it is essential to report this to your doctor immediately. Most of the time, your GP will give you a substitute medication upon consultation, but do not discontinue any medication that you are having right now if there is still no official advice. Bad habits, especially smoking, are another common cause of erection problems. Smokers are two times more at risk to suffer from erectile dysfunction than nonsmokers. Nicotine is a substance that constricts blood vessels. And the blood vessels of the penis need to be in the pink of health to achieve strong and prolonged erections.

Alcohol could also suppress your erections. Despite the popular belief that alcoholic drinks like wine or beer can get you in the mood for love, the truth is it actually hinders a man to maintain an erection. Too much alcohol could also lead to hypertension and obesity that often leads to an erection disorder. It stops the arteries from properly dilating thus there is not enough supply of blood carried to the penis. Because of this, the penis cannot attain and sustain the needed erection. Aside from alcohol, if you abuse the intake of amphetamines, barbiturates, cocaine, marijuana, methadone, nicotine, or opiates, this shall affect the central nervous system which then damages your blood vessels and results in chronic erectile dysfunction.

Having a struggling relationship could also affect a man's erection. When a man is always anxious, irritated, or angry, his mind is not able to focus on making love with his partner. Sometimes, it could also mean a gradual loss of fascination or appeal in having sex when in an old relationship. If this is the cause of the dysfunction, then counseling may be a viable treatment option. Chronic stress, over-fatigue, and depression also causes erection issues. It affects the mind, making a person lose interest in having sex altogether. Chronic stress and anxiety disorders are responsible for about 20% of all erectile malfunction issues, and they are more common in younger men.

With that, below are eight of the most powerful and effective erectile dysfunction cures.

Test Yourself - 6 Questions

How do you know whether your inability to maintain or get an erection is a mental or a physical issue? Answer the following questions to find out...

1. During masturbation, HOW DIFFICULT is it to maintain your erection untilejaculation?

2. During sexual intercourse, HOW OFTEN were you able to maintain yourerection following penetration?

3. When you attempted sexual intercourse, HOW OFTEN was it satisfactory foryou?

4. When you had erections with sexual stimulation, HOW OFTEN were yourerections hard enough for penetration (entering your partner)?

5. How do you rate your confidence that you could get and keep an erection?

6. During sexual intercourse, HOW DIFFICULT was it to maintain your erectionto completion of intercourse?

Did you notice a pattern? I am not a doctor and this is not a diagnosis, but common sense tells me that when you can easily get an erection during masturbation, you the problem is not one of physical nature.

Just keep what you've answered here in mind as you continue reading.

Must Know: Types, Symptoms, and Risk Factors

The most obvious symptom of erectile dysfunction is the sufferer's inability to have and keep an erection long enough to enjoy a sexual activity. It is different from premature ejaculation, because in this condition, a man is having difficulty in developing an erection at all.

An individual can have problems in having full erections from time to time, or slowly becoming frequent, or regularly. Experiencing it occasionally is usually a sign that the problem is not so serious and the individual may only need more rest. While developing it slowly can be a sign of another disease that is causing it, such as heart disease, diabetes, or multiple sclerosis. If it is very frequent, then you need to consult with your doctor right away. There are many types of erectile dysfunction, but they can generally be classified into two: physiological and psychological. Physiological erectile dysfunction is typically caused by an underlying physical disease or illness, while a psychological erectile dysfunction has something to do with the mind. Around 80% to 90% of erectile dysfunctions are physiological in nature.

Males with diseases that affect the arteries, heart, kidneys, and liver are at greater risk of acquiring erectile dysfunction. Other risk factors are drug abuse, obesity, riding bicycles, smoking, stress, and surgery. The usual risk factor is age because when you grow older, your body does not release as much testosterone as it did before which then lessens your overall sexual desire. (Tip: Watch out for my bonus!)

Your body is not as active as before with the presence of more fat, hypertension, and higher cholesterol which contribute to suffering from ED. Men aged 50 and older are also prone to ED but there are males in their 70s and 80s who still enjoy an active sex life.

A man's lifestyle can show how vulnerable he is to erectile dysfunction. Couch potatoes, smokers, alcoholics, and drug abusers are twice as likely to experience erection disorders even at a younger age. Adapting to a healthier lifestyle change can improve erection problems by a lot. Here are some tips on how to do it:

Have more physical activity . Office workers who are stuck inside their cubicles from 9 to 5 are more prone to having erection issues because of their lengthy sitting time. The penis needs sufficient blood flow and healthy nerves and arteries to keep an erection. Sitting for long durations damages that. Stand up every 15 to 30 minutes to stretch and walk around even inside your cubicle for a little while. Perform some body weight exercises or cardio such as jogging in place and jumping jacks within your work area for a few minutes to improve blood circulation.

Furthermore, you should walk whenever possible . For example, park your car at the farthest spot from your office building so you can walk for a bit. If you can take the stairs instead of the elevator, then do it. This will help you increase your physical activity throughout the day even if you are stuck in the four corners of your workspace for eight hours. Maintain your ideal weight. Being overweight or obese contributes a lot to erection problems. In essence, erectile dysfunction is usually just a sign of a more serious disease. Penile erections rely heavily on a healthy cardiovascular system, and medical conditions that damage it, such as diabetes, hypertension, and heart diseases are usually the main culprits.

Other than that, obesity promotes snoring and other sleeping disorders that cause daytime tiredness, lethargy, and melancholy. This excessive tiredness results in lack of sexual interest in the long run. Obesity directly lowers the testosterone and libido levels as well. Consult with your doctor on what is the best way to reduce weight down to your ideal level and how to maintain it.

Reduce alcohol intake. If you are an alcoholic, then get professional help and treatment immediately. It is good not only for your erection issues, but also for your life as well. If you only drink occasionally, then limit yourself to one bottle of beer, or one glass of wine, or one shot of liquor every time.

Quit smoking. This is perhaps one of the most effective ways to prevent and cure erectile dysfunction, but is also one of the hardest. The best approach is to stop it gradually. Choose a date about two weeks to a month away and gradually cut down the number of sticks you are consuming. List down all your triggers and try to be mindful of them. Stay away from areas or places that remind you of smoking. Ask for the support of your family and friends to help you stick to your commitment. Replace your smoking habit with a healthier and productive one, such as running, reading, writing, or cooking.

On your schedule day to quit, throw all cigarettes and smoking paraphernalia away and out of sight. Keep yourself busy with your newfound habits and continue to stay away from places that prompt you to smoke.

Do not abuse drugs. Illegal drug use is another perpetrator of erectile dysfunction. Ask your family and loved ones to help you get immediate professional help if you are already addicted.

2. Food and Diet

Unhealthy food intake could also trigger erectile dysfunction so it is important to know the foods that cause it, and which ones promote a healthier penile function. It is not surprising that the advice of medical experts is the same on how to maintain an overall fit body and how to foster a healthy penile erection.

Eat a healthy and balanced diet. A diet plan that includes more vegetables, fruits, fish, whole grains, and fresh foods prevents and cures erectile dysfunction effectively. In contrast, foods that have excessive fat, sugar, salt, and alcohol, especially processed foods, are the main contributors of erectile disorders.

In connection with some of the above information, a balanced diet helps you reduce weight and fight off obesity, which as you already know causes a lot of other serious medical problems. One study revealed that men who have a waistline of 42 inches and above have a 50% more chance of developing erectile problems than men who have a waistline of 32 inches and below.

Eating a healthy diet also strengthen your body's cardiovascular system, which is central in preventing penile woes. Lowering down your cholesterol, blood sugar, and triglyceride levels is effective in curing any erection issues.

Below are some foods that help prevent and cure erectile dysfunction:

Dark, leafy, and green vegetables. These are great natural sources of zinc, which increases sperm health and testosterone and libido levels. Experts suggest that zinc inadequacy in the body is one of the principal causes of erectile dysfunction.

Nuts. Almonds, peanuts, and other types of nuts are so high in Vitamin E, which helps in maintaining strong arteries and veins.

Watermelon. Aside from being rich in vitamins A and C, this fruit also contains large amounts of citrulline. Citrulline is an amino acid that relaxes blood vessels and strengthens the erectile tissues of the penis. The highest concentration of citrulline is in the watermelon's rind. You can slice a small part of its rind and combine it with its flesh and some ice in a blender to produce a healthy and tasty shake.

Chocolates. One particular food that promotes a solid and dependable erection is chocolate. Cocoa is rich in nitric oxide and flavonoids, which strengthen and enhance cardiovascular health. Dark chocolates are the best because they improve blood flow and increase the amount of nitric oxide in the blood.

Chicken, salmon, lamb, beef, and turkey. These proteins are also high in zinc that, as mentioned earlier, improves testosterone levels and sperm potency. Garlic is also known to fight ED because it increases the body's level of hydrogen sulfide and it has allicin. Hydrogen sulfide relaxes the arteries and blood vessels while allicin boosts blood circulation. They both enhance the circulation of blood to your penis.

Indian and Chinese physicians use garlic as an aphrodisiac and they combine a tablespoon of it with a tablespoon of honey thrice daily. Onions are second to garlic in terms of enhancing sexual capability.

You can also combine a couple of lemons with their peel, two to three tablespoons of honey, and a cup each of dried apricots, prunes, seasoned raisins, and walnuts. Take a teaspoon of this mixture thrice daily one hour prior to each meal. This will help you have and maintain an erection.

You can also dice three medium-sized onions to be soaked for ten minutes in half a liter of lukewarm water. You should then take a hundred millimeters of this thrice daily to get an erection.

Drinking coconut water shall also help you with erectile dysfunction as it has electrolytes like magnesium, potassium, and sodium. These electrolytes promote a healthy contraction of the muscles which in turn assist fluids such as blood to flow through your body, particularly the penis.

Aside from being flavorful, spicy foods can help boost your libido and make you have a satisfying sex life. They urge your heart to drive blood through your body. They also allow the blood vessels to expand and these help get blood to your penis' tip thus causing an erection.

Increasing blood flow is the consumption of foods enriched with jalapenos and chili peppers. Stay away from consuming a lot of peppers, though, as they irritate the bowels and stomach.

3. Herbal Supplements

One of the most popular erectile dysfunction cures today are herbal supplements. They are used by many people around the world not only for their acclaimed usefulness for improving sexual potency, but also for many other known health benefits. Some of the most well-known plant supplements for sexual disorders are ginkgo biloba, saw palmetto extract, panax ginseng, and yohimbe.

Ginkgo biloba - this supplement comes from the leaves of a tree with the same name. It is indigenous to China and is an essential part of traditional Chinese medicine. Ginkgo biloba is popular as an aphrodisiac and has highly positive effects when it comes to fortifying vascular nerves and tissues. It acts as a powerful antioxidant as well. Other benefits of this herb are for improving cognitive performance, enhancing blood flow, and managing hypertension, multiple sclerosis, and clinical depression.

Saw palmetto extract - this supplement is an extract from the fruits of the saw palmetto palm tree. Aside from being known as a sexual enhancer, this extract is also touted as highly effective in alleviating the symptoms of benign enlargement of the prostate (BEP). Because it basically shrinks the prostate's mass, it loosens that penile arteries which promotes a good erection. Its use have originated from early American Indians, which utilized the herbs for treating urinary tract infections and other reproductive system disorders. The extract's other uses are for relieving headache, colds, coughs, asthma, sore throat, bronchitis, and some flu-like symptoms.

Panax ginseng - also known as Korean Red Ginseng, this herbal supplement used to treat and manage a number of mental and emotional conditions, such as chronic stress, clinical depression, anxiety disorder, and daytime fatigue. Aside from being a common treatment for erectile dysfunction, some males also use it to manage premature ejaculation. Other medical benefits from this herb are cancer prevention (including skin, lung, liver, breast, and ovarian cancers), cure for diabetes, gastritis, anemia, and asthma, and for strengthening nerves, joints, and vascular tissues.

Yohimbe - an herbal supplement made from the bark of an African evergreen tree of the same name. It contains a chemical called yohimbine that some experts claim is an effective cure for erectile dysfunction.

It is important to note that the herbal supplements mentioned above are not regulated, and you are at risk of experiencing some side effects when using them. Yohimbe can be dangerous to your kidneys and heart when taken in large amounts, while panax ginseng is known to cause insomnia and other sleeping disorders to its users.

The United States Food and Drug Administration (USFDA) also does not endorse their use, but you may still consume them at your own risk. In order to ensure your safety, consult with your local health practitioner first before using these products. The Chinese have used for centuries the herb ginseng for addressing the problems of low libido and erectile dysfunction. This herb improves blood circulation throughout the body and boosts the production of testosterone. It also improves your mood and aids in treating erectile dysfunction due to non-physical causes.

Another herb that can help reverse erectile dysfunction is yohimbe from the African yohimbe tree's bark. This herb has been utilized since the ancient times to increase libido and treat erectile dysfunction. The extract called Yohimbine comes from yohimbe which you can obtain only if you have a prescription, but it can reverse erectile dysfunction.

Gingko biloba helps boost blood circulation as well as raise the blood oxygen levels. It also frees the blood vessels of obstructions and enhances memory and concentration.

For many centuries, Ayurvedic health professionals have used the herb saw palmetto to treat erectile dysfunction and improve the reproductive systems of males. It is very effective in lowering symptoms of prostate that is enlarged, a condition affecting flow of pelvic blood and increasing chances of ED. This herb is available in extract or pill form.

Chinese herbalists usually mix other herbs such as stinging nettle with saw palmetto berry to come up with a blend that can fight erectile dysfunction. Such herbs can be combined with honey to be consumed as tea or paste.

Erectile dysfunction can sometimes be due to an infection and this can lead to damage or inflammation of the mechanisms needed for an erection. One of the antifungal herbs that are so effective is tea tree oil which can be applied topically. You should dilute this and then use to wash your genital area. This oil treats infections that cause problems such as inflammation which have a bad effect on your erectile health.

It increases the activity of white blood cells in the spots where it is applied. You can actually use this to cure infections which may cause ED. The herb ashwagandha root reverses erectile dysfunction as this boosts sexual energy. It reduces stress and strengthens your immune system. Its extract has anti-inflammatory effects that lower prostate inflammation and heighten sexual health. As mentioned earlier, vascular health is vital to achieve erectile health as this increases your general sexual health.

Vascular health is very important in achieving erectile health because it is needed to ensure sufficient blood flow to your penis. When you suffer from inflammation of the prostate, this affects the flow of blood to your vascular area which could have otherwise helped in ensuring a good erection. When you minimize prostate inflammation, this will boost blood flow to your pelvic region. The herb guduchi stem contains anti-inflammatory properties and an antitoxin. It is also anaphrodisiac that treats erectile dysfunction. You should consume two grams of guduchi stem in dried powder form twice or thrice daily to treat male impotence.

By now you should've discovered the secret: Drop the processed food, eliminate fast food and replace all that with a balanced, healthy diet full of fresh, organic vegetables, legumes and fruits. That will not only help you cure ED or make your erection even stronger; it'll make you feel good and enjoy life at a higher level!

4. Vitamins

Aside from having the proper diet and taking herbal supplements, vitamin supplements can also prevent and treat erectile dysfunction. Below are the essential vitamins needed to improve your erections:

Vitamin A - this is a very important vitamin in terms of regulating progesterone. Progesterone is the most essential progestogen hormone of the human body. One of its many functions is stimulating the sexual drive of an individual (both male and female). And for a male person, it can help in treating erectile problems.

Foods rich in Vitamin A: green, leafy vegetables, yellow fruits, squash, fish, milk.

Vitamin B - most of the complex B vitamins are able to give positive effects when it comes to penile erection. Vitamin B1, or thiamin, strengthens nerves and vascular organs that helps improve penile functions. It also provides more energy all throughout the day which can translate into more energy during sexual intercourse as well. Vitamin B3, or niacin, stimulates the body's systems to produce more sex hormones and improves the cardiovascular system as well. Meanwhile, vitamin B9, or folic acid, helps increase sperm count and potency, which leads to more lengthy erections. Vitamin B12, or cobalamin, is another vitamin that strengthens the nerves and blood cells of the body.

Foods rich in Vitamin B: pork, liver, carrots, oatmeal (B1); mushrooms, eggs, (B3); pasta, bread, cereals (B9); and meat and other animal dairy products like milk and cheese (B12).

Vitamin C - apart from helping your body create more sex hormones and boosting your sperm count, vitamin C also strengthens your vascular nerves, arteries, veins, and capillaries for better blood flow. An added benefit is that it helps lower bad cholesterol and increase stored energy, which will not only make your erection last longer during intercourse, but your performance as well.

Foods rich in Vitamin C: citrus fruits, tomatoes, guava, cabbage, chili peppers, red bell pepper, green bell pepper, cauliflower.

Vitamin D - a recent study at the University of Milan in Italy regarding sexual disorders reported that insufficient supply of vitamin D in the body can lead to an erectile dysfunction. The study revealed that all of the men that had erection problems have 20% lesser amounts of vitamin D in their systems as compared to those who have natural erections. They have also found out that vitamin D is responsible in maximizing the use of nitric oxide in the body. And nitric oxide stimulates the vascular muscles to relax, making them more open so blood can flow efficiently. And you know that when blood is flowing freely and efficiently, erections are more intense as well.

Foods rich in Vitamin D: Mushrooms, liver, fish, egg yolks, cheese.

Vitamin E - this vitamin is a powerful antioxidant, which, like vitamin D, helps stimulate the circulation of nitric oxide in the body. Aside from helping your body fight cancer cells from multiplying and decreasing your risk of having heart attacks, vitamin E can help you with your penile issues as well. It also stimulates the production of prostaglandins, which are powerful hormones that increase libido.

Foods rich in Vitamin E include: almonds, raw seeds, hazelnuts, kale, spinach.

Other nutrients that help improve erectile problems:

Zinc - as already mentioned above, zinc improves the potency of sperm cells, and it increases testosterone and libido levels too. A 250 mg supplement a day can help you a lot if you have erection problems.

Foods rich in zinc include: oysters, shellfish, nuts, chicken, salmon, lamb, beef, and turkey.

Omega-3 fatty acids - a healthier and stronger heart leads to a more productive sex life and penile erection as well. And omega-3 fatty acids helps a lot with regards to preserving your heart. It also increases the generation of nitric oxide in the body.

Foods rich in omega-3 fatty acids include: salmon, tuna, vegetable oils, soybean, flaxseeds, kale, spinach.

Selenium - around half of selenium in a man's body is found in his testicles and semen canals. If he is suffering from selenium insufficiency, then chances are that he will suffer from erectile dysfunction as well.

Foods rich in selenium include: brown rice, chia seeds, Brazil nuts, shitake mushrooms, broccoli, spinach.

Magnesium - this trace mineral is responsible for producing estrogen, androgen, and brain chemicals that is responsible for boosting libido levels. If you are low on this, then it will be difficult for your penis to have an erection.

Foods rich in magnesium include: leafy vegetables, avocado, fish, beans, whole grains, nuts, seeds, bananas, dark chocolate.

5. Exercise

As mentioned in the first item of this list that incorporating more physical activity in your daily life could do a lot to improve your erection problems. In addition, having regular and consistent exercise is definitely an important physical activity to put into your schedule if you want to achieve that.

A 30-minute brisk walk every day is actually enough to lower your risk of suffering from erectile dysfunction by 40%, so you don't have to start with something so complex or unrealistic. After that, you can gradually increase the intensity of your daily workouts as your body gets used to it. You may even add strength training eventually. This will further lower your risk of having erectile issues. The good news is that when you start to experience the benefits of having regular exercise in your schedule, you will naturally want more and will then benefit more.

Researches also show that moderate exercise can cure erectile disorders from middle-aged obese men if done consistently. British health experts have suggested performing Kegel workouts (which enhances the pelvic muscles) to boost penile function.

Exercise will also allow you to maintain your ideal weight, which is another great way to prevent premature erectile disorders.

Professor Wayne Hellstrom, an urologist from New Orleans' Tulane University School of Medicine, revealed that the penis is "a barometer of what's happening in the rest of the body." This means that when you have an erection problem, this usually means that there is a more serious medical condition that you are suffering from, such as a heart disease or diabetes. And he said that exercise is a key component to recuperate. Also know that continuous exercise boosts the function of the endothelium, which is the inner lining of the blood vessels. When the endothelium is healthy, blood flows freely and smoothly all around the body. Exercise is a great way to deal with erectile dysfunction.

As you get older, your body becomes easily sore. Therefore, you do not have much time to exercise. Because of this, you allow your body to degrade a bit by gaining weight and becoming out of shape. It can be so difficult to get back to proper shape so you may find yourself not even bothering to do so. Because of this, the blood flowing throughout your body decreases and this can cause erectile dysfunction.

Among the best exercises are cardiovascular workouts such as walking, running, jogging, and swimming. You can even perform jumping jacks so that blood will continuously flow through your body, particularly to your penis. (If you can't see yourself doing any of this think about how you could modify it to make it more appealing. Listening to music while jogging, or watching TV while you're on the treadmill, etc.)

Pelvic contraction is another exercise to help reverse erectile dysfunction. It is very simple to perform and it begins with lying on your back on a comfortable surface as you do not want to hurt your back while you exercise. Lie on a cushion or blanket for comfort if you will lie on the ground. Bend the knees apart with the feet staying flat on the floor.

Tighten the pelvic muscles which are closest to the ground and perform this strongly and fast. Hold the muscles for ten seconds and then relax for another ten seconds after loosening the muscles. Perform three sets of this exercise two times a day.

One of the best yoga exercises which promote blood circulation through the pelvis is the lying pump. If you are not in good shape, this can be hard to do. Begin by lying on the floor and then breathing evenly and deeply throughout the workout. This is vital to achieve the proper effect. Push the small of your back against the floor so as not to strain the lower back.

Inhale and exhale and then lift the right leg gradually as you inhale. Hold this for five breaths. While you exhale, lower the leg. Your breaths will set the pace of the workout. Do this exercise on the left leg and repeat the whole exercise ten times.

You can also perform squats as these build your legs' muscle mass and increases the blood flow to the lower body. If there is more blood flow to the groin, this shall provide more energy to the lower area so you will avoid suffering from erectile dysfunction again. To perform a squat, place your hands on your waist and then bend the knees outward.

Your back must be kept straight and then lower yourself to the floor as close and as comfortable as you can. Never strain your body. Perform five to ten repetitions of this daily.

Another exercise is by sitting on a chair with your back straight and not resting against this chair. Inhale deeply and then raise the testicles through the contraction of the pelvic muscles. Hold this position for as long as possible but not more than ten seconds. Once you have relaxed, take a rest for ten seconds. Do such contractions two times daily. This workout produces good results when you do them with pelvic floor contractions.

6. Yoga

The introduction of this article said that around 50% of erectile dysfunction sufferers are under the age of 75. Some of them are still in their middle years. Gone were the days when erection issues are only experienced by old men. There are many reasons why this is happening, and some of them are: more stressful work environment abundance of processed foods that leads to nutrient deficiencies new medications for different chronic illnesses like clinical depression and diabetes smoking and alcoholism

These things are more common in middle-aged men. One of the newest treatments used for erectile dysfunction these days, particularly those of middleaged sufferers, is yoga. Yoga is a Hindu exercise or discipline that focuses on developing a person's physical, mental, and spiritual life aspects. Typically, it includes distinct poses or stances, breathing exercises, and meditation. Its main goals is to bring happiness, wellbeing, strength, and relaxation to the practitioner.

Yoga practitioners believe that a person's health is mainly based on the health of his own life force. When his life force is low, then his health will also be low. Yoga lifts a person's life force up, and with it is his wellbeing as well. Physically, the stances, meditation, and breathing exercises of Yoga relax the body's nerves, arteries, and veins, which allow blood to circulate more smoothly around the body.

7. Homeopathic Medicines

The use of homeopathic medicines to cure erectile dysfunctions are also becoming popular these days. Homeopathy is an alternative cure that is based on the concept that "like cures like". It was discovered in 1796 by a German scientist named Samuel Hahnemann. While some people believe that homeopathy is pseudoscience, there were many confirmed accounts of its effectiveness for the last two centuries.

What makes homeopathy appealing is that its medicines all come from natural substances and not artificially or chemically processed. Homeopathic medicines work by energizing and boosting the body's own self-healing capacities. Homeopathy experts claim that it provides permanent cure to erectile disorders and that it treats the condition from its source and does not only help the patient alleviate its symptoms. Its practitioners also believe in the presence of an individual's life force (similar to yoga), and that when it is affected, it affects a person's overall wellbeing.

Thus homeopathic medicine targets not only the physiology of a patient, but also his mental, emotional, and spiritual aspects. This means that utilizing homeopathic treatments heals your whole being - body, soul, and spirit - taking away physical illnesses, psychological disorders, and spiritual problems as a whole. When you use homeopathy to treat your erection problems, your own body is actually treating itself. The medicine simply lifts your body's self-healing abilities to make it faster.

8. Hypnotherapy

Finally, another new method of treatment for erectile dysfunction is hypnotherapy or hypnosis. Hypnotherapy is a kind of psychotherapy that involves establishing transformation or change in the subconscious mind of a sufferer. It involves videos, music, or a combination of both with a voice-over narration.

Hypnotherapy is only effective if the cause of an erectile dysfunction in a man is psychological in nature. Some of the most common psychological causes of erection problems are chronic work-related stress, financial problems, relationship or marital issues, sexual anxiety (worrying about having an erection actually hinders erection), guilt, clinical depression, feelings of self-pity and self-inadequacy, and loss of sexual interest in your partner.

Listening or watching hypnotherapy music and videos cure psychological erectile dysfunction and low sex drive by: reestablishing your influence and selfcontrol over your sex drive through your subconscious mind, lowering any feelings of worry, guilt, and indifference with regards to your own sexual abilities, restoring the impulsive and instinctive human response to sexual arousal, and restoring the appeal, excitement, and carnality of having sexual intercourse. Hypnosis allows you to uncover subconscious sexual obstructions that hinder long-lasting erections. It also allows you to create new beliefs and connections with regards to sexual intercourse or making love, which build up your own self-esteem and self-confidence that you can satisfy your partner.

Many website today offer this kind of service for treating erectile disorders. A quick search on the internet will readily lead you into one.

Medical Disclaimer

It is advisable for you to consult your doctor and know why you are suffering from erectile dysfunction. You have to find out if there is a physical cause which your physician would be able to determine. He would then be able to suggest natural remedies to make you have and maintain a solid erection. If these natural cures do not work, ask your physician if you can take medications such as Cialis, Levitra or Viagra. They treat male erectile dysfunction and are proven effective against many causes as long as you do not suffer from hypotension, uncontrolled hypertension, or diabetes. If these are not ideal for you, ask your doctor if you can take alprostadil.

This is a self-administered medication in the form of either a penile suppository or injection. This medication increases the flow of blood to your penis for you to have and maintain a strong erection. A penis pump is for you if you are not comfortable with using medications for erectile dysfunction. This is a battery or hand-operated device which utilizes a vacuum and a constriction band or ring for you to have and maintain an erection. You use this device for half an hour at a time. While the band or ring is in place, you can have sexual intercourse because of a solid erection.

If all these fail, it may be necessary for you to undergo surgery. There are two options for this. If your ED is due to poor blood circulation, you may need vascular surgery as it removes blockages. Another option is a penile implant in your penis which may be inflated for you to have an erection at any time.

The Perils of PORN

The modern man has a lot of sexual stimulation, even if he does not have a sexual partner. The sex industry has become a huge part of our economy, and this was initially protested for the basic reason that it went against the morality of religion. A big part of this sex industry is pornography. With the advent of the internet, pornography became far more easily accessible, which meant that the number of people that watched porn on a regular basis went up dramatically towards the end of the twentieth century.

Although pornography is no longer protested against on religious grounds (in most parts of the world at least) it is having a significant impact on male sexual health. Since porn is now so widely accessible, it has become very easy to get sexual stimulation. As a result, a lot of people have started to become addicted to porn. This is not common enough to warrant concern about the legality of pornography, however the overuse of this medium of sexual entertainment is one of the possible causes for erectile dysfunction for a number of reasons. Some of these reasons are as follows:

Pornography is Not Real

When you look at pornography, you are looking at something that is at best an idealized version of actual sex and at worst is something that is purely artificial and has been made in order to attract a large number of plays and views. However, the major concern here is that by watching porn you are cutting the intimacy out of your sexual relationships. This means that you get used to sexual release without having to deal with emotions later. You get used to sexual situations where you do not have the responsibility of pleasing anyone but yourself.

This results in the formation of a sexual dynamic within your mind. In this sexual dynamic, you are the center of sexual attention in your world. Hence, when you enter into an actual sexual encounter, the pressure you are under may end up being something that you just cannot handle. As a result, you begin to panic. The presence of someone beside you ends up being a factor that adds greatly to your stress during sex. Since you have become so used to sex that is not real, that has been skewed for the purpose of garnering as many plays as possible, you end up unable to deal with the real thing.

Pornography Can Result in Disconnection

As has been stated before, when you watch porn you achieve sexual gratification without the emotions that ensue following sex. As a result, you are unable to deal with real emotions during your actual sex life. Healthy sex involves as few partners as possible, because having sex results in emotional bonding and doing that with too many people is just not healthy. However, if you are a regular watcher of porn, you may end up being unable to deal with emotions at all.

The major effect that this will have on your sex life is that it will cause a great deal of strife as far as emotions go. You will be simply unable to provide that emotional connection for your sex partner, and as a result your relationship will suffer. Due to this emotional disconnect, you just would not feel aroused during sex because you fear the aftermath. You will end up dreading having to face connection with somebody as you will be completely not used to such a thing, and erectile dysfunction will ensue.

You Get Used to Masturbation

If you have enjoyed both sex and masturbation, you will know that, although both activities end in the same result, they are completely different if you really understand them. With masturbation, the pressure you apply is much greater and you are in control of how much pleasure you feel. However, a vagina cannot apply the same amount of pressure, and while you are thrusting you cannot control your own pleasure the way you would with your hand.

Masturbation is not harmful in any way whatsoever, it is the overuse of it that might end up harming your sex life. When you masturbate, you get used to that specific type of sexual gratification. The end result is that your sex life suffers. When you are used to pleasing yourself you are unable to feel the same pleasure that you would feel if you were less used to masturbation.

This where the stress comes in. Keep in mind that stress is one of the most important factors that can go into erectile dysfunction. Hence, the stress that comes from not enjoying sex as much as you think you may very well end up causing you erectile dysfunction. There are several other ways in which masturbation can affect your sex life as well. One of the major ways is that you do not understand how to please your partner during sex. Masturbation is by definition a solo affair, and while masturbating the only thing that is on your mind is your own orgasm.

You get used to instant gratification while masturbating regularly, and watching porn is an important contributing factor to this dynamic, particularly due to the fact that women in porn conform to the dynamic that men are the only ones who should be pleased in porn. Real sex requires a more long term approach, so to speak, as women require more time than men to climax. Hence, if you are just trying to achieve orgasm yourself while having sex, you can be sure that the woman you are having sex with is not going to enjoy having sex with you.

Not satisfying your sexual partner during sex will end up increasing the amount of pressure you are under during sex. You are going to end up feeling unsatisfied with your own sexual prowess and this will result in major stress that will eventually end up in erectile dysfunction. One of the most significant ways in which masturbation can affect your sex life is by disrupting the flow of testosterone in your body. Healthy masturbation habits are actually good for your testosterone. Masturbation keeps everything functioning smoothly as it were, and whenever you have an orgasm your testicles end up producing more testosterone because they are so heavily stimulated.

The problems start to occur when you start masturbating too much. Once you start masturbating twice or more a day, your body would be put under a fair amount of strain. If you are masturbating so much, your testicles will be heavily focused on replenishing your sperm count. Usually, if you are masturbating within a reasonable amount such as four to six times a week, your testicles are easily able to replenish your sperm count. As a result, the other functions that your testicles are responsible for, such as the production of testosterone, are not interrupted and continue as normal.

However, masturbating too much means that your testicles end up working overtime in order to replenish your sperm count. As a result, they get overworked and stop producing as much testosterone as they should. This can result in low levels of testosterone in your body overall. Testosterone is important for libido, as it is the very hormone that makes men male. Hence, having low levels of the stuff in your body can result in erectile dysfunction or low sexual arousal.

Too much of anything is bad, and the same goes for masturbation as well. You might just be causing your body to lose out on testosterone, which might end up causing your erectile dysfunction. Avoiding masturbation for a period of time is a good way to gauge whether this particular type of erectile dysfunction is what you are suffering from.

Pornography Gives You Unrealistic Expectations

This is possibly one of the most significant drawbacks of watching pornography. When you see pornography, you are seeing something that has been processed for the purpose of consumption. The women you see have been carefully picked as have the men. Additionally, most porn involves a great deal of makeup and post production in order to make the actors and actresses seem absolutely flawless because that is what ends up selling and getting the most views. Most people realize that this is not real life that is being shown in pornography, and expecting this level of perfection in real life is unrealistic.

However, when your only source of sexual gratification is porn, you get used to seeing unimaginably beautiful women and men. As a result, when you see people who are real, people with actual flaws, you end up getting disgusted by this, or at the very least have a problem getting aroused. The problem with the idealized world of pornography is that even the actors don't really look like that. Were you to see pictures of adult actors, you would find them completely unrecognizable. However, while watching porn you don't realize this and come to see the way they look as natural.

This will eventually make it difficult for you to get properly aroused while having real sex. All you will be wondering is why the person you are having sex with does not look like the women you were fantasizing about having sex with for so long. This is one of the major causes of erectile dysfunction as far as porn is concerned. When the real thing does not fit your idealized fantasies regarding it, you will be disappointed and will be unable to arouse yourself without some kind of depiction of said fantasy.

Another way that porn can cause erectile dysfunction is by giving you unrealistic expectations about the sex itself. Sex in porn caters to your fantasies, and is not generally a depiction of how sex is in real life. In general sex in pornography is designed to be visually and aesthetically appealing. The problem here is that real women generally would not like to have sex the way it is shown in porn. They will probably enjoy watching it the way you do, but the fact remains that they would not enjoy the roughness of sex in porn, and would require a much subtler and more delicate touch.

In pornography, people change positions several times over the course of sex. These positions are often uncomfortable for the woman. In real sex, however, building up sexual pleasure within a single position is more common. Additionally, women are treated as sex objects in porn. Some women do enjoy this in real life, but at the same time a lot of women might not and you will have to respect that. By watching porn you would get used to the idea that women like being treated this way and that would contribute to problems in your sex life.

As a result, there will be constant dissatisfaction in your sex life. You will essentially be a selfish lover, and the lack of satisfaction your partner would be getting from sex would end up putting pressure on you. As you already know quite well, when pressure or stress comes into it erectile dysfunction is only another step away. The inability to satisfy your partner, despite having sex exactly the way they show it in porn, would result in you being unable to get erect during sex because you will fear that you will disappoint your partner.

Porn doesn't just give you unrealistic expectations regarding sex and the woman you are having sex with. It also gives you unrealistic expectations about yourself as well. The actors in porn are usually muscular ubermensch with very large penises. You, on the other hand, probably would not be as genetically gifted as these porn stars. This is generally of no concern, as women generally have realistic expectations of the men in their lives. As long as you are reasonably fit, something which is quite easy to achieve, you will be quite attractive to women because personality tends to be more important than looks.

Additionally average penis size is actually smaller than you might think. As long as your penis is around five and a half inches while erect, you have a penis that is of comparable size to any other adult human male. This is actually very important for women. Most women simply cannot take a penis that is larger than around six and a half to seven inches at the most, and this is the extreme limit as far as vagina capacity is concerned. Penises that are larger than this could end up causing damage, and even penises that are extremely large in size but fit can cause discomfort during sex.

This is why most women tend to avoid men with extremely large penises in real life. Having sex with a man with a large penis tends to be an uncomfortable ordeal for most women, so if you have an average sized penis you are actually more likely to have sex than if you had an enormous penis that was made for porn. All of these realities are thrown out in the window for porn, however. In pornography, women love only men with huge muscles, and they only have sex with men who have huge penises.

In porn, women are shown to derive pleasure from huge penises. Size matters only in porn, but in these videos women are shown to absolutely love a man that is well endowed. From all that you have read, you know that this is completely untrue. Most porn actresses look at these scenes with men who are well endowed to be challenges that have to be overcome. They look at such scenes as uncomfortable, but necessary in order to do their job right.

However, if the only way you receive sexual gratification is through pornography, then you might not realize this. You might look at your average male body and your average sized penis and think that these things are inadequate in some way. After all, in your major sexual experiences you have only seen penises that are at the very least seven inches long. As a result, you might end up feeling inadequate during sex. You would feel that the woman you are having sex with does not enjoy the way you look, and would be under pressure to behave in the way that most male porn actors behave.

Since you do not conform to the beauty standards that have been set by porn, you might end up getting erectile dysfunction as a result. The main cause is the inadequacy you would feel, and there is no real way to get over this if you are still watching porn on a regular basis. If this is a major problem for you, it is important to realize that there are such things as sexual chemistry. Women need sex just as much as men do, and just as you might find women attractive even though they don't look like porn stars, a lot of women will definitely find you attractive as well.

Porn Causes Escalation

You might start off by watching regular porn. Just the sight of a woman without her clothes would be enough to get you fully aroused and achieve climax when you first started watching it. However, you don't last long at this level.

Eventually, you get so used to seeing videos of women without their clothes that you end up needing more and more to get you going. This is not your fault. As human beings we are bound to get bored by doing too much of anything, which is probably why you would start watching porn that is increasingly "more" of something or the other.

Most people go the route of violence. When regular porn no longer gives them the buzz they desire, they start craving porn that is more extreme in some way. Porn in which women are put in pain or dominated, porn that involves extreme levels of sexuality. This simply because these men are starting to get desensitized to sex. By watching so much porn, you will have made it so that the sight of a woman with her clothes off is something commonplace, something you see every day. Not to mention the fact that the women in porn are enhanced surgically as well as through makeup and post production editing and effects.

Eventually you will want porn that is more "active", in which there is more screaming or more positions or something else extreme. You will want more no matter what. The problem here is that most of this cannot translate into your sex life. Some women will not like choking, others won't like being slapped around. You will have to conform to some extent to your partners sexual needs and restrictions.

You might not enjoy having sex the way it is shown in pornography yourself. You might not enjoy treating women like sexual objects, you might not like morally bereft and emotionally disconnected sex. However, you might be conditioned into thinking that this is the only real way to have sex, because you will have watched so much porn in which this is the norm. Hence, when your real sex life does not correspond to this norm that you have appropriated watching stylized and fictional depictions of sex, you will end up feeling emotionally empty, uninterested in real sex and erectile dysfunction will ensue.

Porn escalates without us even knowing it. The progression occurs in minute steps but can occur in a short period of time. Hence, within no time you might be watching porn that has rape in it, porn in which acts of extreme violence are conducted against women. These are not healthy sexual preferences at all, and chances are they are not your sexual preferences either. You have just become so desensitized to regular porn that you are no longer able to get aroused by it, which is why you are satisfying yourself instead by watching porn that is increasingly violence, increasingly excessive and all in all distasteful.

How To Quit Porn Forever

If you have a porn addiction and it is causing erectile dysfunction, the best thing to do is to quit it completely. Porn addiction is no different from addiction to alcohol or drugs, it can cause major disruption to your life and since it involves an area of your life that is extremely intimate and linked to your overall happiness it can be considered even more dangerous.

Since addiction to alcohol and drugs is treated by absolutely abstaining from whatever you are addicted to, the same must apply to porn. However, this is easier said than done. If you are addicted to porn, how are you supposed to quit it?

Here is a list of techniques you can use:

Accept Your Addiction

This is an incredibly important first step that you must take. Without acceptance, there is no chance that you will ever get over your porn addiction. This is most commonly done in the form of an affirmation. You need to say to yourself, "I am addicted to porn." It would be more effective to do this in front of a mirror, since this way you are going to be able to see yourself saying it.

Get Someone Involved

Doing it all on your own is not possible. You need to be answerable to someone about your habits. Since you are trying to quit porn completely, it is important that you have someone who is inquiring about your daily activities. Think of this person as a sponsor. If you are feeling like watching porn, you can at least have someone to talk to who will talk you out of it. Someone that might end up providing an alternative. This can even start an intense romantic relationship for you.

Block Access to Porn

You can do this by using a number of apps. Just make it as difficult as possible for you to watch porn online. By using a parental app that allows you to block certain websites, you can ensure that you will be simply unable to watch porn at all. It is important that you enlist the aid of your friend in this. Blocking certain sites requires you to create a password, a password that you should not know. Have your friend create this password and keep it a secret from you, so that you have absolutely no way to bypass the app.

Remove Any Porn that is in Your Personal Possession

One of the biggest signs that you are addicted to porn is that you have a "porn collection". This is acceptable only if you have never been addicted to porn. If you are serious about getting over your addiction, you need to destroy every piece of porn that is in your possession. That includes DVDs, magazines and any pornographic files that you might have stored on your computer. Once you have destroyed and deleted everything, you will have no choice but to conform to your new lifestyle choice.

Disable Internet Access for a While

This is a rather extreme measure that you should only take if your porn addiction has gone out of control. In order to be safe from the dangers that pornography poses to you, you should disable your access to the internet completely for a while. This might end up keeping you safe from any temptation to watch porn entirely. If you don't have internet to waste your time with, you can fill your days with more positive activities, activities that are healthier and can help you get over your addiction and have a more positive sex life.

Get Help from a Professional

Sexology is a growing field, and there are a number of people in this field who would be able to address your addiction and help you get over it. In order to beat an addiction that has spiraled out of control, professional help might end up becoming necessary. The benefit of enlisting the help of a professional is that you no longer have to worry about doing it all yourself or putting strain on a friend or someone you love. Instead, you can unload and vent to someone who is being paid to listen.

Keep a Diary or Journal

When you write your thoughts down, you transform them from subjective pieces of your psyche to actual objects that can be analyzed objectively without the biases of your own mind. By writing down whenever you want to watch porn, you will be able to transform your addiction into something manageable, something that you can see with an objective eye. It becomes a tangible thing instead of a terrible addiction that has taken hold of your mind. Doing this is one of the most effective ways to get over your addiction.

Whenever you feel the need to watch porn, just write down what it was that made you feel this way. This is called identifying your triggers. You will either see that the thing that made you so aroused is not something you are supposed to be aroused by, or you will recognize it as a genuine threat to your "sobriety" and would be able to avoid it in the future. You might even recognize that not all of your triggers are sexual in nature. Some triggers might be things like stress, which would mean that your porn addiction is just another way to cope with stress which is very understandable.

Keeping a journal such as this is also a great way to write down your feelings about sex and how you feel about having erectile dysfunction. As you already know, much of erectile dysfunction is about stress. By writing down the things that stress you out, you are going to become more in control of how you feel.

Great Alternatives To Porn

One of the best ways to get over your porn addiction is to find alternatives. Some of these are sexual some are just distractions to keep your body busy, but all of them are excellent ways to quite porn.

Exercise

Exercise is a great way to get the blood pumping. What you need to realize is that exercise gets blood pumping to whatever muscle you are working out. First and foremost, this distracts you from whatever it is that is making you want to watch porn. Exercise is a great way to relieve stress, which is one of the primary reasons for addiction in all cases. Additionally, by exercising you are going to fill up your time. When you don't have time for porn, you will find that the addiction will fade away entirely. It doesn't help that you are going to become much more physically fit as a result!

Exercise can also help with erectile dysfunction in general. By boosting blood flow within the body, exercise makes it easier for your body to get blood to your penis. Slow blood circulation is one of the biggest reasons for erectile dysfunction, so tackling this issue can make it much easier for you to get over your problems getting erect. Create a short exercise routine (no more than ten minutes long) that you follow whenever you have the need to watch porn.

Meditate

Meditation is an excellent solution for anyone that is suffering from porn addiction. By calming your internal storm, you will make it easier on yourself to get over your need for porn.

The meditation technique you should use involves deep breathing and a calm, collected seated pose. Sit in a place where there is nobody around you, somewhere secluded. Ensure that while you are meditating you are bathed in as much natural light as possible. If you are meditating at night, do so in the dark as it will be better than drowning yourself in artificial light. Once you are seated in a room with natural light or darkness, whichever you prefer, take deep breaths while counting to four, holding for just a second, and then exhale while counting to four.

You will be amazed at how much this calms you down. If you want your meditation to be more effective, you can make it so by focusing on a single point. Close your eyes, imagine a ball of light surrounded by pitch darkness and focus on it. This will give you an alternative to pornography that will calm you down and preserve your sobriety. It is also a great way to handle stress.

Alternative Ways to Masturbate

As long as you don't masturbate to porn, doing so is not discouraged while recovering from a porn addiction. You will find that the reason you were masturbating so much was the fact that you were watching porn, and once you have stopped watching it you will want to masturbate a normal, healthy amount.

However, what are you going to masturbate to? You can't watch porn, but you can fantasize about things. Fantasies are a perfectly legitimate way to masturbate and get aroused because they are personal and are not affecting your personality in any way. It is also a very good idea to write down your fantasies. Remember, writing things down makes them real. This means that when you write your fantasies you can make them tangible and thus more erotic. It will also help you ascertain whether your fantasies are reasonable or not.

Having fantasies locked up in your head leaves them out of your ability to judge them objectively. However, putting them on paper allows you to examine them as if they were objects rather than parts of your conscious mind. Additionally, you can start using erotica as an alternative to porn. Erotica contains erotic content by nature, and can provide you with a healthy way to masturbate and arouse yourself. The benefit of erotica is that it is usually written for a unisex audience. This means that the content of the erotica that you will be reading is not going to conform to the unhealthy standards of beauty and sexual practice that are provided by pornography.

Moreover, since erotica is meant to be read rather than passively watched, it can encourage you to form a more positive body image and also have more realistic expectations of what women will look like since you will be projecting the women you see day to day as the characters in the erotic novel rather than idealized, airbrushed and surgically enhanced porn stars. Another benefit that erotica provides is that it often describes sex in a more accurate manner, or at least a manner that would be more suitable to what a woman would want during sex. As a result, you will learn how sex can be something pleasurable for both of you rather than something that is solely for your own pleasure as is posited by pornography.

Sexting and Phone Sex

If you find it difficult to get aroused during actual sex, you might find sexting and phone sex more to your liking. This is because sexting provides you with a image based form of sexual gratification which is close to what you are experiencing with pornography. Phone sex also takes a lot of pressure off of you since it does not require you to do much else than last long enough on your own to allow your partner to satisfy themselves. Since you will be masturbating on the phone, and masturbating is what you are used to at this point, you will not be faced with what is in your current opinion an inferior form of sexual gratification, since it does not provide the same level of pressure and control, and would thus have no problems engaging in sexual activity.

Another important technique you can use is video calling. This gets your sexual experiences as close to pornography as possible. Engaging in such activities will allow you to bridge the gap between actual sex and pornography, thus making it easier for you to engage in sex later on in your relationship. Essentially, you will be replacing pornography with an analogue that is more conducive to a stable relationship and mutual sexual gratification.

Prostate Gland

Stress is certainly a major cause of erectile dysfunction, but it is certainly not the only cause. Sometimes erectile dysfunction is caused by biological malfunctions in your own body. One of these malfunctions has to do with the prostate gland. One of the most common reasons for erectile dysfunctions is prostate cancer. In this chapter, potential ways to stave off prostate cancer will be discussed. A technique called prostate massage will also be discussed in detail.

What Causes Prostate Cancer?

Unfortunately, it is not quite clear what causes prostate cancer. Apart from bad genes that cause you to become predisposed to cancerous cells in that region, it is unclear whether lifestyle has any impact on your risk of getting prostate cancer.

What is known is that prostate cancer is caused by abnormal behavior of the cells in the prostate. A mutation in the cell will cause it to replicate itself more quickly than it needs to, which results in the surrounding cells that are replicating at a normal rate to start dying. This is what results in an enlarged prostate. It is one of the most significant biological causes of erectile dysfunction. Despite the fact that the causes of prostate cancer are not known, it does affect a fair number of men every year. Six out of every hundred men will get prostate cancer before the age of seventy. Hence, if you are worried about your erectile dysfunction, go get a prostate exam done. Your troubles in bed may be caused by either prostate cancer, or some other irregularity in your prostate. Getting it checked before it gets serious will help you avoid major problems later on.

How To Prevent Prostate Cancer

Eat Foods that are Red

The best food in this category is the tomato. The reason these foods are so good for you is that they are chock full of antioxidants which, as you probably know quite well, are very good for you. As far as tomatoes and other red fruits go, the particular antioxidant that they possess which will be particularly useful for you is called lycopene. This antioxidant has been scientifically proven to be able to prevent the growth of cancerous cells in your prostate, or anywhere else in your body.

This is not to say that if you start eating a kilo of tomatoes a day you will not get cancer. If you are predisposed to cancer because of your genes, no amount of food will help. However, consuming lycopene rich foods can certainly help you to postpone cancer, or at least make it less likely to happen. It is recommended that you cook the red foods that you are eating. This makes the lycopene easier to digest for your body. Additionally, try your hardest to ensure that the red foods you do eat are really as red as they can possibly be. The redder they are, the more lycopene that they will have in them.

Stock Up on Green Foods

Green vegetables are also a great option for you if you are looking to reduce the risk of getting cancer. Green vegetables contain a variety of different nutrients, all of which can be very beneficial for you if you are at risk of cancer. These nutrients contain compounds that help destroy carcinogens. If you are looking for a single set of entities that cause cancer, carcinogens are it.

Thus, by stocking up on green vegetables, you will ensure that your body has enough chemicals that can help fight carcinogens, thus making it less likely for you to get prostate cancer. It is highly recommended that the vegetables you eat are as fresh as possible. This means that the majority of your vegetables should come in the form of green salads. Try not to pile on dressing, as this will make the process by which your body would be extracting nutrients from these green vegetables less efficient. Remember, these vegetables need to become part of your diet. They are not medicines that you can temporarily take and then stop when you feel like your health has improved.

Avoid Junk Foods

Sometimes, it not so much about what you add to your diet as much as it is about what you remove from it. A lot of the foods that you eat are terrible for you, and you might be surprised to learn that many of them might end up causing cancer in the long run. This is because a lot of fast foods and junk foods contain carcinogens. This is because of the process by which they are cooked. Deep frying and other such cooking techniques that create unhealthy, fattening foods also flood these foods with carcinogens.

Hence, the more junk food and fast food you eat, the more likely you are to get cancer in the long run. It is important that you realize that there really is no acceptable level of junk food or fast food consumption. Every time you eat fast food, you are making yourself more liable to get cancer. Therefore, the best option is to simply cut the fast food out entirely. Replace the fast foods with leafy greens and red foods and you will make it very unlikely for yourself to ever get prostate cancer.

Eat as Much Fish as You Can

Fish is really a miracle food. If you must eat meat, make sure that the meat you eat the most is fish, as it is the healthiest of all of the meats. Many would consider it to be the tastiest as well! A lot of people tend to avoid fish claiming that it is fattening. However, it is the very fattening properties that people criticize about fish that make it so effective at preventing all forms of cancer, especially prostate cancer.

The fatty acids that are within fish are no regular fatty acids. They are omega-3 fatty acids. This particular type of fat is actually very similar to lycopene, with only a few minor differences in its chemical structure that classify it as a fat molecule rather than an antioxidant. This means that by eating fish, you are going to flood your body with omega 3 fatty acids, and this is going to severely reduce your chances of getting prostate cancer. It is important that you do not fry the fish you eat. By doing so, you are leaching out the precious nutrients you are eating it for, and might even end up filling it with dangerous carcinogens.

Eat Tofu and Other Soybean Products

Tofu has long been a darling of vegans everywhere. This is because it is widely considered to be an excellent meat analogue. It is made from soybean, and as it turns out soybean, as well as other foods such as chickpeas and peanuts, contain a chemical that is very effective at combating cancer. These particles are called isoflavones, and they are notable because they specifically make it less likely for you to get prostate cancer. It is unknown why this particular chemical is able to reduce the risk of prostate cancer, but the results don't lie and they are what you should go on.

Even if ou have cut out fast foods and junk foods from your diet completely, you are not nearly out of the woods yet. This is because of a rather sad fact about the diet of modern man. In our diet, we consume massive amounts of fat. Whether it is in the form of the substance we cook our food in, meaning practically every kind of cooking oil, or the substance that we use to accompany practically every food we eat, such as butter or cheese, fat has become an irreplaceable part of our diet.

This is dangerous because a high consumption of fat has been consistently linked with a high rate of prostate cancer. Hence, if you want to avoid prostate cancer, and the inevitable erectile dysfunction it brings, you will have to cut fat out of your diet. You can do this by replacing the butter or fatty oils you use with olive oil. Additionally, you can opt for healthier snacks such as celery and raisins instead of fatty snacks such as chips of French fries. By making such replacements, you are going to make it far less likely that you are going to get prostate cancer.

Smoking is a habit that is absolutely terrible for your health in every way. Although smoking is commonly linked with lung cancer, it turns out that smoking makes you more likely to get every type of cancer. This means that if you smoke, you forty percent more likely to get prostate cancer, especially if this particular type of cancer runs in your family. Additionally, if you are recovering from prostate cancer, smoking will actually cause you to relapse rather quickly. A lot of people think that quitting smoking is impossible difficult, but doing so is actually a lot easier than it seems.

If you smoke, give nicotine gum a try. It is a great way to satisfy your nicotine craving without having to pollute your body with toxins that would end up causing cancer. You can quit at any time in your life. Within ten years of quitting, your life expectancy will have returned to that of a non smoker, so no matter how old you are give quitting a try and make it less likely for you to get prostate cancer.

Folate is in a lot of foods that you eat, and you might not realize just how much of it you are actually eating. This is because folate is not widely considered to be a harmful food. So much focus is put on fats and other such chemicals that folate seems to get ignored. However, it has been scientifically proven that consuming too much folate may result in an increased risk in cancer. Although it is certainly not as bad as eating fatty foods or smoking, avoiding folate rich foods may just push you over the edge of the boundary wall that surrounds the people that won't get prostate cancer!

Several foods that are actually considered healthy contain folate, such as oranges. Do not cut these foods from your diet completely. Instead, cut them down, and don't eat more than is absolutely necessary. Try to create a diet plan in which you ascertain how much of each food you are going to eat. Additionally, avoid all supplements that contain folic acid. The majority of vitamin supplements actually contain this chemical, so be very careful. Folic acid is required in only the tiniest of trace amounts, and excess consumption could lead to prostate cancer.

Take Adequate Amounts of Exercise

A buildup of fat is one of the main causes of prostate cancer. Weak muscles also end up making the prostate work more than it is supposed to, which ends up making the prostate go into overdrive by multiplying cells faster than it needs to, thereby leading to prostate cancer. Lucky for you, there is a single solution that solves both problems simultaneously: exercise. By taking exercise you are going to reduce the amount of fat in your body in vast amounts, and you are also going to strengthen your muscles.

You don't necessarily have to go to the gym to get adequate exercise. Just try to take up a sport, or try to go running every day. Even if you don't take out time specifically for exercise each day, there are ways in which you can incorporate exercise into your daily routine. For example, you can take the stairs instead of using the elevator. You can also try walking more, especially if your office is close by. Try eschewing cars for public transport, as this mode of transportation inevitably requires you to walk more.

Get Regular Checkups

The key to prevention is to getting to know as much as you can about your physical health. Get regular checkups done and keep your doctor in the loop about your physical health. Doctors can often predict very early signs of problems in your prostate, which can help you to alter your lifestyle in order to delay the inevitable cancer as much as possible. Additionally, doctors can help you out a lot by prescribing medication that can help you keep your prostate healthy. Often, when you are suffering from erectile dysfunction, once you start taking prostate medication your dysfunction will disappear completely.

Your doctor can also tell you about telltale signs of prostate cancer. This will allow you to skip the regular checkup as long as you know what you are looking for. By recognizing the symptoms early on, you will be able to go to your doctor immediately and have him or her check you out properly. All in all, visiting the doctor is the best thing you can do if you are trying to prevent prostate cancer.

Giving Yourself A Prostate Massage

In order to promote the health of your prostate, you can engage in prostate massages. These can be done by a medical professional, but this is not necessary. You can definitely do these massages yourself. Here are the benefits of performing prostate massages:

You Can Discover Cancer Early On One of the biggest signs of cancer is an enlarged prostate. If you ever go to the doctor, he will probably perform something akin to a prostate massage in order to ascertain whether your prostate is enlarged in any way. However, going to the doctor requires a fair bit of hassle on your part. Attending regular checkups can become a stressful affair, especially if you have a busy work life.

Additionally, having someone else perform a prostate exam on you is a distinctly uncomfortable affair. After all, someone you don't even know is going to have their fingers up your posterior. By performing prostate massages, you can discover any abnormalities in your prostate right at home without having to worry about taking time out of your schedule. It certainly doesn't hurt that prostate massages can also be an excellent way to boost your pleasure during sex, or that they can become sexual practices in and of themselves, which is something that is going to be discussed in the next chapter.

It Helps Drain Seminal Fluid

One of the major causes of erectile dysfunction actually has nothing to do with prostate cancer itself. Rather, it has to do with one of the more significant causes of prostate cancer, thereby occurring in the buildup to the cancer itself.

Often, a buildup of seminal fluid occurs. This fluid collects within the passage it takes to your penis every time you have an orgasm, as not all of the fluid is drained out of your penis when you climax. As this fluid builds up, it starts putting immense amounts of pressure on your prostate. Once the buildup becomes severe, it can cause your prostate to get inflamed. As a result, your testosterone levels become imbalanced, thereby resulting in erectile dysfunction.

If you give yourself regular prostate massages, you will find that the seminal fluid will not be given the opportunity to build up. This is because whenever you give your prostate massage, you will be draining this seminal fluid. During the massage, the fluid will be ejected from your body via your penis. This is a great way to prevent prostate inflammation altogether, thereby greatly reducing your chances of prostate cancer. You can also use this technique to help you if you are suffering from erectile dysfunction, regardless of whether you are afraid of getting cancer or not.

It Relaxes the Prostate

Another major reason that the prostate could be causing erectile dysfunction is that a lifetime of stress and tension often results in tightened and tense nerve endings and muscles around the prostate. This is because during our flight or fight response we tend to clench all of our muscles, the muscles surrounding our prostate glands receiving some of the most intense pressure of all. As it turns out, we experience our fight or flight response quite a bit, despite the fact that we are no longer hunted by carnivorous predators.

Now such reactions occur in board rooms and conferences where you are put under the spotlight. Since you do not have a direct face of danger that you can either fight or flee, your muscles do not experience the same kind of relief that they would if the danger you had faced was more tangible, something that your body could actually handle. When these muscles receive so much pressure on a constant basis, they tend to become used to being so tight. As a result, they adopt a tense position permanently. This ends up damaging the nerve endings that surround the prostate too.

Keep in mind that this is a very sensitive part of your musculature. When you have a fight or flight response to something, it is the muscles in your anus, the ones coincidentally directly connected to your prostate, which get clenched first. Hence, taking care of this tension is not just recommended, it is necessary. When the area surrounding your prostate is suffering from so much tension and strain, your prostate gets damaged as a result. It stops functioning normally, and your body gets less testosterone than it should. One of the biggest things that it causes is erectile dysfunction.

By massaging your prostate, you are going to relieve the nerve endings and muscles that surround your prostate. When you do so, you are going to bring your prostate back to its normal state, where it can function the way it is supposed to. Hence, if you are suffering from erectile dysfunction, ask yourself if you have been under a lot of stress recently. Chances are, a prostate massage can relieve some of the stress and help you get erect once again.

Prostate Massages Stimulate the Prostate Gland

A lack of testosterone results in many problems for males. Low facial and body hair, an inability to gain muscle, and, perhaps the most sinister of all, erectile dysfunction are all problems that are caused by a low amount of testosterone in the body.

The prostate gland is one of the primary sources of testosterone. Sometimes you are just naturally predisposed to having a low amount of testosterone in your body. This is genetic and is not the result of your lifestyle. Other times, your lifestyle, such as a poor diet or lack of exercise, would result in your prostate becoming inefficient and producing testosterone. Either way, the end result is the same. You already know how important it is to change your diet and get more exercise if you are suffering from erectile dysfunction. You can also use prostate massages to increase testosterone levels in your body.

When you apply pressure to your prostate, you stimulate it. This actually causes a fair amount of pleasure. You are feeling this pleasure because your prostate is starting to release more testosterone. This is a natural result of stimulation and pressure. Massaging any gland in the body will make it secrete more of its specific hormone. Hence, if you feel like your testosterone levels are low, give yourself regular prostate massages. You can even have your partner do it and make your sex life kinkier and more exciting!

It Improves Blood Flow to the Prostate

One of the biggest reasons that your prostate could be causing erectile dysfunction is that it is getting an inadequate amount of nutrients and oxygen. The main reason for this is that your body is not directing enough blood to that area of the body, as blood is the liquid that transports nutrients and oxygen to the various parts of your body. It is important to notice here that your prostate is in the same general area as your penis. As a result, low blood flow to the prostate mean low blood flow to the penis as well. You can see how the two are connected now. Low blood flow to your groin in general can cause erectile dysfunction. Hence, your inability to get erect may be caused by your prostate being malnourished, or low blood flow to your groin. Both of these problems can be fixed via a prostate massage.

It is a natural part of our biology that whenever we stimulate or massage a certain part of our body, the blood vessels in this part of the body will dilate, thereby improving the flow of blood in that particular area. When you massage your prostate, you are improving blood flow in your groin, because blood will have to flow through their to get to your prostate. In this way, your penis will have more blood to help engorge it and make it erect. Additionally, your prostate will have a steady supply of oxygen and nutrients to keep it healthy, thus preventing erectile dysfunction from that end as well.

It Cleanses the Prostate

Over the course of your life, every part of your body gets collectively impure. This is because the majority of the food we tend to eat is full of chemicals and germs that infect our body, assaulting our organs. Mineral buildups are common, as are blockages and such caused by bacteria.

Your prostate is similarly susceptible to buildups of bodies that will cause it to become, for all intents and purposes, "dirty". A dirty prostate is clogged up and unable to perform basic tasks such as the production of testosterone. You have probably altered your diet by now, meaning that you have stopped the flow of impurities to various parts of your body, including your prostate. However, the impurities that have built up in that area already are still there, and your body is going to take a long time getting them cleaned out.

You can expedite the process using a prostate massage. By massaging your prostate, you will force it to eject the impurities that it possesses into your blood stream, thereby cleaning it out and making it resume production of testosterone at full capacity once again. If you have not changed your diet, prostate massages become a regular requirement. Since your body is still being filled up being impure and unhealthy foods, your prostate is going to suffer from a buildup of impurities frequently, thereby requiring you to clean it out with the same frequency lest you start suffering from erectile dysfunction again.

Prostate Massage is a Good Substitute for Masturbation

Often, people who suffer from erectile dysfunction are unable to masturbate. This is just an inevitable part of one's inability to get erect. If your erectile dysfunction is caused by biological imperfections rather than stress or the fact that you are too used to masturbating and pleasuring yourself to enjoy sex properly, being unable to masturbate is a legitimate concern. Luckily, you have prostate massages to save the day. Prostate massages can remove the urge to masturbate in two ways. Firstly, these massages are quite pleasurable. In fact, a lot of people say that orgasms induced by prostate massages, and they certainly are possible, are more intense and pleasurable than regular orgasms.

Secondly, prostate massages remove excess sexual desire. Since you are regulating the flow of testosterone in your body, you will be less likely to suffer from spike is in testosterone levels. As a result, you will no longer suffer from the sudden bursts of sexual desire that you might have gotten used to by now. By using prostate massages, you will be able to at the very least make up for your lack of an erection. Just remember, erectile dysfunction does not make you any less of a man. It is just a disorder you are suffering from, and prostate massages are just a way to get over this disorder. Do not think of it as something you have to do because you can't get erect.

Prostate Massages Help Reduce Prostate Inflammation

Prostate Massages Help Reduce Prostate Inflammation

There are myriad causes for prostate enlargement. However, prostate enlargement has a single major end result: prostate cancer. If your prostate remains enlarged for too long, it will inevitably result in cancer, and throughout the time it is enlarged you are going to suffer from erectile dysfunction. By using prostate massages, you will be able to address this inflammation. If your inflammation and swelling is not the result of cancer already, or if you are not genetically predisposed to getting cancer, prostate massages can help to prevent your inflammation from ever evolving into cancer at all.

This is because prostate massages help to soothe that part of your body, boosting blood flow and nutrient flow to it. As a result, your prostate is not going to have to work as hard to do its job, which is going to help it remain healthy. Remember, an overworked prostate will inevitably get inflamed. Prostate massages are also a great way to keep cancer at bay even if you are genetically predisposed to it. It can also negate some of the effects of cancer to a small extent. This is because you are helping your prostate fight off the cancerous cells. It is certainly not in any way guaranteed to cure you, but the fact remains that it can certainly prove to be a useful supplement to your chemotherapy or whatever medical alternative your doctor is providing.

It Stimulates an Increase in Seminal Fluid and Sperm Count

Seminal fluid is something that your prostate plays an important role in creating. Your sperm is your testicles designated job, but the testosterone that your prostate provides is what gives your testicles the ability to make sperm in the first place.

As it turns out, both seminal fluid and sperm have a role to play in erectile dysfunction. Or rather, a lack of either or both could be the cause of your erectile dysfunction. Testicular massages are mostly erotic in nature and do not really have an effect on sperm count. However, prostate massages increase the flow of testosterone in your body. As a result, your sperm count is going to increase because your testicles will have more material with which they can create sperm. They would be less overworked as well, as the whole process becomes easier with an adequate amount of testosterone.

Additionally, prostate massages allow your body to produce more seminal fluid. You may have noticed that right after sex or masturbation, it takes you a fairly long time before you can climax again. This is because your body requires seminal fluid in order to feel aroused. Hence, a low supply of seminal fluid is a major cause of erectile dysfunction. By stimulating your prostate gland, you are going to increase the amount of seminal fluid, thereby making it far easier for you to get aroused and erect. Additionally, you will notice that you will be able to have sex more often after performing these massages on yourself regularly.

It Makes it Easier to Urinate

One of the biggest side effects of a swollen prostate is difficult urinating. This mostly because of the location that the prostate gland can be found in. The prostate gland is generally found behind the scrotum, pressed up against the rectal wall. Hence, when the prostate gland is swollen, it tends to press against the urethra. The urethra is where your urine flows from. If your prostate is enlarged, it will narrow that passageway, thereby making it far more difficult for you to urinate. This can cause severe discomfort, as you will feel the need to urinate but will be unable to do so. The urinating process can also become painful for you.

By stimulating your prostate gland, you are going to make it a lot easier for you to urinate. This is because you are going to be directing blood flow to your prostate and reducing inflammation. Once the inflammation has been reduced, your urethra will no longer be blocked and you will be able to urinate freely. Prostate cancer can also help you if you have started to urinate while asleep. This is also caused by irregularities in your prostate that are affecting your urethra. When you massage your prostate, you are going to remove these irregularities and thus vastly reduce your chances of urinating in bed.

Prostate Massages Make Sex Better

Prostate massages are great at helping you boost your libido. Once your libido is up, you are going to want to have sex more often, and thanks to the increased amounts of seminal fluid in your body you are going to be able to have sex again sooner after climaxing without having to worry about sudden drops in passion or your penis suddenly going flaccid while you are having sex.

Additionally, prostate massages open you up to a new world of pleasure in your orgasms. This because oftentimes we are unable to fully enjoy our orgasms because impurities in our prostate prevent us from reaching those levels of ecstasy. This is why when you massage your prostate and clean it out you are going to notice that your orgasms are a lot more intense.

Massaging your prostate will also help you to stay hard for longer. You will essentially be able to hold out for a longer period of time before climaxing, thereby allowing you to satisfy your partner as well. This helps if you have a tendency to climax before a lot of stimulation, and can only last a minute or two in bed. In this sense, prostate massages can also be a great help for people who suffer from premature ejaculation. With so many widespread benefits of prostate massage, what are you waiting for? There are absolutely no drawbacks whatsoever, so there are no negatives for the positives to outweigh.

Enjoying Sex In Spite of Erectile Dysfunction

Just because you have erectile dysfunction doesn't mean you can't enjoy sex. There are a lot of people out there who enjoy full and happy sex lives despite the fact that they suffer from erectile dysfunction. In fact, there are a lot of people that can go their entire lives suffering from erectile dysfunction and not have any major problems with their sex lives. There are a number of activities you and your partner can do in order to enjoy sex and intimacy together that won't put pressure on you to get erect.

Mutual Masturbation

One of the biggest reasons that you might be suffering from erectile dysfunction is that you are too used to masturbating on your own. The vagina would not be an adequate tool for getting you erect because you just don't find it as pleasurable as the firm grip of your own hand. When you masturbate, you tend to know exactly what to do in order to have a pleasurable experience. It's your body after all. Hence, the orgasms you feel when you masturbate would appear to be a lot more intense than the one's you'd be feeling with your partner.

However, this does not mean that you cannot be intimate with your partner and masturbate at the same time. Masturbation is a great way to enjoy each other's bodies. Usually when you masturbate you probably think of someone, a fantasy or something similar. You might watch porn. By masturbating with your partner you are going to be able to enjoy each other's bodies while masturbating. Your partner might just prefer this if she is a woman. Just like woman don't quite know how men like to be touched, men don't know how women like it either. By masturbating in front of each other you can achieve intimacy without having to have intercourse.

You can also use mutual masturbation as a way to get erect before having sex. Try progressing to this level if you want to eventually be able to have penetrative sex with your partner. It is highly recommended that you at least try to penetrate your partner once you are erect. Another way you can use mutual masturbation to progress to sex is by masturbating your partner with your own fingers. Have her guide your movements, telling you where to go and what to do. By doing this, you are going to discover her body and where her pleasure lies. It is going to add a significant amount of intimacy to your relationship because you are going to be the one giving her pleasure.

Additionally, you can create a sexual connection by having your partner help you masturbate. You can guide her hands yourself, as this will teach her how to properly give you pleasure. It will at least be a step above simply looking at and touching each other while masturbating, and is an important stepping stone to getting over your erectile dysfunction. You and your partner can also make the experience more erotic by rubbing lube or oil on each other. Once you have gotten yourself hard, have your partner put oil or lubricant on your penis for you. This has the added benefit of getting you used to her touch as well, which will make it easier to have sex later on.

You don't have to try to do this the very first time you and your partner are intimate. However, in the long run mutual masturbation should really be considered as a buildup to penetrative sex. This is because penetrative sex is the most intimate form of sex there can be. If you are unable to have it you are not deficient in any way, but you might be missing out on sex that is truly transcendent.

Use Sex Toys

Sometimes, your partner just needs some sexual satisfaction from you rather than from themselves. It is a perfectly ordinary request, and fair considering they are a sexual being too. Hence, it is important to give you partner sexual pleasure using whatever tools you can. A great way to do this would be to use sex toys. Sex toys are great because they can actually substitute for your penis in a lot of ways, and in certain ways can even provide superior pleasure.

There are several sex toys that you could use in order to get your partner off. The most popular is probably a vibrator. By using a vibrator, you will be able to provide intense pleasure to your woman. By applying it to your woman's clitoris, you are going to be able to give her intense orgasms. The use of vibrators is extremely effective, and is actually a normal sexual practice. It is a misconception that woman derive pleasure from penetration. While there is an erotic quality to this act and penetration does indeed provide a great deal of pleasure, most women find it extremely difficult to achieve an orgasm while they are being penetrated.

This is because a woman's pleasure center is actually outside her vagina: the clitoris. Hence, even if you and your partner were having penetrative sex, you might still be using a vibrator to get her off. That's just the way things work sometimes! However, this does not mean that your use of the vibrator on her has to be restricted to her clitoris. You can use the vibrator in a variety of other ways. One very popular use of the vibrator is on her G spot.

Her G spot is located inside her vagina. It is actually roughly in the same part of her body as your prostate is in your own body. Hence, if you are familiar with prostate massages, you are going to have no trouble whatsoever discovering this part of her body. If you use the vibrator on her G spot, you are going to be able to give her truly incredible orgasms. Indeed, her orgasms will be far more pleasurable than they would ever have been had you been using your penis instead of a vibrator. This is because a vibrator provides the stimulation of intense vibration aside from the thrusting motion that you are using it for.

If you want to get really kinky you can use two vibrators at the same time. One can be used on her clitoris, and the other one can be used on her G spot. By using two vibrators at once you are going to give her orgasms like she has never felt before! There is a cornucopia of other sex toys that you can use as well. One great example is an anal plug. By putting an anal plug into your partners anus, you can provide intense stimulation to her. The act is intensely erotic and also tends to feel quite naughty as does anything that has to do with the anus.

A great sex toy that you can use is a string of anal beads. These are a series of beads that are either strung together or form a single plastic rod. You will insert these beads into your partner's anus and use a vibrator on her clitoris. Once she is climaxing, you can pull the beads out of her anus to push her orgasms to another level entirely! You can also use vibrators and anal beads on yourself. Remember, your prostate is extremely sensitive, and by stimulating it you can induce powerful orgasms within yourself.

You must use thinner vibrators than you would be using on your partner's vagina. Having your partner do it for you can make the experience a lot more erotic, and will probably end up giving even more powerful orgasms than you were expecting to have. You can also use anal beads on yourself while you are masturbating. Simply masturbate in front of your partner and have her keep a finger on the beads. Once you are about to achieve climax, have her pull the beads out in one movement. This is going to stimulate your prostate intensely. You are going to feel a sudden shock to the prostate with each bead that brushes up against it.

This can help you to enjoy far more stimulating orgasms. Additionally, your partner will be involved in the process of giving you pleasure. This is extremely important. Sometimes your partner would want to be the one who is giving you pleasure. It just feels good to know that the pleasure is coming from something one is doing to one's partner. By involving your partner in this way you will be able to enjoy sex together. Additionally, if you are in a same sex relationship, anal beads can become a great way for you and your partner to enjoy each other's bodies. You can use vibrators on each other as well in order to bring intimacy to the sex. Hence, by using sex toys you will be able to have excellent sex without having to get erect at all.

Sexting and Phone Sex

This is a great way to keep sex in your lives even if the two of you are extremely busy. It is important to keep the sex alive even if you are unable to meet each other. By using your cell phones you can create a level of deep intimacy before having to actually get down to having sex. This is quite important, because having actual sex may be a very stressful experience for you. When you get into bed with a new partner, you might be under a lot of pressure to perform. You already know what pressure does to someone suffering from erectile dysfunction.

As a result of this pressure, it is going to be absolutely impossible for you to get erect during this first encounter. The best thing to do if this is the case is to "soften the blow" as it were.

By engaging in sexting and phone sex you are going to get used to your partner's sexual preferences and body without having to be under pressure to perform for her. Since you are simply getting images while sexting, getting hard won't be a problem for you if the erectile dysfunction you are suffering from is not severe and caused by biological anomalies. Sexting, hence, is the very first tier of gaining intimacy. Once you and your partner have sexted a little, you can move onto phone sex. Phone sex is a great way to take your intimacy to the next level. This is because you can actually hear each other's voices, and will be able to see the effect you are having on each other.

You can also respond to what your partner wants you to do. You might be asked to send a picture of yourself, or your partner might ask you to engage in a fantasy with her. This will allow you to gain a deeper understanding of her sexual preferences. You can use phone sex to discuss your own sexual preferences as well. One very important thing that phone sex might be able to help with is actually talking to your partner about your erectile dysfunction. Since you are going to be able to discuss it in a safe space of your choosing, and if your partner's responses are not what you expected you can always cut the call, discussing it over the phone is a great way to break the news without having to go through the stress of a face to face conversation about something so embarrassing.

Once the two of you have gained an adequate level of intimacy, you can move onto some more advanced levels of virtual sex. This would be video calling. Phone sex is great, but after a certain point you need to be able to see your partner respond to your sexual preferences and requests. You would want to be able to actually see your partner doing what you tell them to, and your partner would most likely want the same from you too. By having sex over a video call, you can attain a much higher level of intimacy. There is only so much you can ascertain from a person's voice. Sometimes, movement is necessary to determine whether what you are doing is in line with what that person wants.

Seeing your partner move while pleasuring themselves is important because it allows you to align your own movements to theirs. The visual component of sex will facilitate a deeper understanding of each other's sexual natures, and is a lot more enjoyable from a purely hedonistic aspect. You can even start incorporating some of the previously mentioned techniques. Sex over a video call is already pretty close to mutual masturbation. You can take this to the next level by incorporating sex toys into it. By having your partner use sex toys on herself, you can give her increased pleasure by proxy.

There are a lot of sex toys that you can use that will bridge the digital divide between you two. Certain sex toys and vibrators come with apps that allow them to be remotely accessed. Hence, you can be sitting in the comfort of your own home and giving your partner intense pleasure over a video call. This does not just remove the need for an erection, it makes the entire process of meeting each other unnecessary for a time. You can save the actual sex for later, while enjoying each other with through a screen for a period of time. Bear in mind that video calling is a big step up from phone sex. With video calling, a lot of the masks you might be able to wear while having phone sex will be gone. You will, literally, naked in front of your partner, or at least in a situation where your partner will be able to see you.

This involves a level of vulnerability that you might not be ready for. You might video call your partner and be unable to get erect, in spite of the fact that you were fully able to over phone sex. There is no shame in this, it is just a natural part of your erectile dysfunction. You are essentially under pressure to perform while on a video call. This is why you will suffer from performance anxiety, which will end up making it very difficult for you to get erect.

Use video sex only when you are ready. Once you start using it, sex practices such as mutual masturbation won't be far behind. You can use sexting, phone sex and video sex as stepping stones to mutual masturbation, which in itself is a stepping stone to getting over your erectile dysfunction and having penetrative sex. You can even use these practices in the gaps between your actual sex encounters. It will help you and your partner to maintain the intimacy you have fought so hard to achieve, despite the fact that you have not met each other in a long time.

Oral Sex

If there is a single sex practice that you should engage in while you are suffering from erectile dysfunction, it is oral sex. This is because it's just a great way for you to give your partner pleasure. The problem with a lot of the aforementioned techniques and methods that you can use is that they involve some kind of barrier between you and your partner. Sexting, phone sex and video sex all involve sex through a digital wall of sorts. Additionally, having sex via mutual masturbation is pretty distant too. You just aren't getting the same level of intimacy you would be getting if you were to have penetrative sex.

Even using sex toys is sometimes not adequate. Although it can provide a great deal of pleasure for you and your partner, using sex toys is still artificial sex. Sometimes your partner would want a more organic touch to the sex you two are having. The best way to bring this touch of realness to your sex life is by engaging in oral sex. Oral sex is far superior to simply touching or masturbating your partner because it involves the use of your tongue. Your tongue is a lot more efficient and getting your woman to climax than your fingers are, probably because of the way it is built. There are several ways in which you can make oral sex a regular part of you and you're partner's sex life.

The key to oral sex is how you use your tongue. You need to press your tongue flat on your partner's clitoris. Make sure it is not flexed or hard. Your partner would enjoy it if your tongue is nice and soft. Once your soft tongue is place flat on your partner's clitoris, you can move it around in circles. This would provide enormous stimulation to the clitoris and would probably result in incredibly intense orgasms. You can get your fingers into it too. While you are giving your partner oral sex, you can penetrate her with your finger as well. Simultaneously stimulating her clitoris with your tongue along with her G spot with your fingers is a great way to give her amazing orgasms. This would be far superior to using vibrators because your partner would be getting her pleasure from an actual part of your body rather than a mechanical object.

A further level of oral sex would be to penetrate your partner's vagina with your tongue. This is rather difficult to do and can be quite uncomfortable for you but it is an intensely erotic experience for your partner for the sole reason that it will show her how committed you are to pleasuring her. The key is to start slow. You don't want to rush into things, and your partner certainly won't appreciate it. Savor her as you pleasure her, she will feel the tenderness with which you are pleasuring her and this will translate into her own pleasure.

It is also important to keep in mind that the clitoris is essentially a female version of a penis. This means that a lot of the things that you find pleasurable, she will also find pleasurable if you do it to her clitoris. Hence, apply some of the techniques that you find enjoyable and you might be surprised at how much she enjoys it. Just remember to try gentler versions of these techniques because a clitoris is vastly more sensitive than your penis. If you really want to get kinky, you can engage in anilingus. This involves stimulating your partner's anus with your tongue. You can just stimulate the edge of her anus and it would provide her with quite intense pleasure. Your partner can even do it to you if you are so inclined!

If you are having sex with a male partner, there are several techniques you can use in order to give him a pleasurable experience with oral sex. A good idea would be to stimulate the head of his penis with your tongue. The head of his penis is home to large cluster of nerves. Hence, is you pleasure this part of his penis, he is going to feel it more intensely than he would otherwise. Try to move your tongue around in a circle around the head of his penis.

If you really want to give him some intense pleasure, you can focus on the area just beneath the head of his penis. This would be the skin that connects the head of his penis to the rest of it. If you gently stimulate this area, he is going to end up having enormously pleasurable orgasms. He might just climax without even realizing he was close, such is the intensity of pleasure he can get from this area. You can also engage in other activities, such as gently stimulating his scrotums with your lips or tongue. This can be very pleasurable for your partner, and would greatly increase the level of intimacy that the two of you enjoy.

One thing you should keep in mind while giving your male partner oral sex is never to get teeth involved. Keep in mind what it's like to receive oral sex yourself. Anything you like is probably going to translate well to him. You can also give anilingus a try with your male partner. This is a very kinky activity and your partner will surely love it just as much as you do. Try rimming the edge of his anus with your tongue whilst simultaneously masturbating him. The twin sensations can result in excellent orgasms for your partner.

All in all, by applying oral sex techniques you can provide your partner with intimate pleasure in spite of your inability to get erect. In fact, a lot of the techniques described here are those that would be used by someone even if they were able to get erect because they are much more effective at providing women pleasure than penetration.

BDSM

BDSM is a great way to bring some spice into your sex life. It is also rather enjoyable for you if you suffer from erectile dysfunction, because if you act dominant to your partner you probably won't even really need to penetrate her. The key here is to communicate. You and your partner should sit down and talk about what you want. If your partner wants you to be submissive, explain to her your sexual dysfunction. It probably won't matter either way, because your partner would want you to be submissive to her and would thus find your erectile dysfunction rather erotic.

There are a variety of ways in which you can spice up your sex life using BDSM techniques. One rather popular way is to use handcuffs. These wouldn't be the uncomfortable variety that police officers would use on convicted felons. Rather, they would fluffier handcuffs, covered in fur to make them comfortable. The fur will also provide a tickling sensation, which will increase your partner's sensitivity in bed. You can also tie your partner up with ropes. Ropes great to use if you want something that will hold, something that will prevent your partner from moving entirely. You will then be able to pleasure her using any of the aforementioned techniques and would thus be able to be in control of the situation.

The benefit here is that you are no longer under pressure to perform. You have your partner entire under your control, and this means that she cannot talk back to you. It is an intensely erotic way to have sex and will probably help a great deal with your erectile dysfunction. Apart from tying her up or otherwise restraining, you can use intense vibrators on her clitoris. While she is tied up, the effect of the vibrator will be much increased. The sensation of being unable to move will increase the intensity of pleasure, and the feeling of the rope will make her more susceptible to even the slightest touch.

One of the best ways to provide her pleasure while she is tied up is to tickle her. This is a form of sexual torture that results in a high level of intimacy. Tickling tends to illicit uncontrolled reactions from the person being tickled. This is why, when you tickle your partner, you are going to end up feeling intense love towards her, and this will help make the sex more intense and enjoyable.

In order to add more spice to your sex with BDSM, you can also blindfold your partner. This will help because it will completely take the pressure off you. She will be unable to see you, and the feeling of being tied up coupled with her temporary blindness will make everything you do to her far more erotic than it is. Even the touch of your breath on her ear will end up making her shudder while she is in this position. Since she is so easy to please while she is like this, you are going to be able to pleasure her without worrying about your performance. You might be surprised to learn about how little your erectile dysfunction matters. When the pressure is relieved, you are going to end up getting hard without realizing it.

You can also engage in submissive behavior in order to alleviate the problems caused by erectile dysfunction. The major benefit of this is that you are not going to be the active participant. Rather, you are going to be submissive to a dominant partner. As a result, she is going to be the one telling you what to do. When the pressure is off your shoulders to perform, when you are put in a situation where the only thing you have to do is follow instructions, you will find that it is a lot easier to get erect than it was before.

You can even encourage your partner to tie you up or handcuff you. Since you will be unable to move and are essentially a passive participant in sex, you will not have to worry about what to do to please your partner. Being in such a passive position makes the whole process of sex much easier for you, and a lot less stressful.

Just keep in mind that you have to communicate each other's desires to one another. Just because you are submissive in bed does not mean that you are in any way less of a man, or that you are somehow supposed to be submissive in every aspect of your life. Sex is supposed to be restricted to the bedroom. Outside of it you can be just as dominant as you have to be. Inside it, however, you can do whatever you need to in order to have sex. While engaging in BDSM, your partner is responsible for your safety if you are a sub. However, this does not mean that you need to keep your mouth shut if your partner is engaging in a sexual practice that you are not comfortable with. If what you are doing or what is being done to you is outside your comfort zone, be sure to tell your partner. Chances are, your partner just does not know that they are crossing a line.

Additionally, being a dominant sexual partner in bed does not mean that you have to cause your partner pain. Whips are a definite part of BDSM, but this does not mean that pain is essential to getting over your erectile dysfunction. Being dominant in bed is not an excuse to hurt your partner either. Sex is always consensual, as is everything that has anything to do with sex. Just remember to keep it safe and to only go to places where both your partners have discussed before. This is primarily a way to get over your erectile dysfunction and allow you and your partner to enjoy sex in spite of the fact that you are unable to get erect.

Masturbating with Your Prostate

If you are experiencing the kind of erectile dysfunction that comes from a faulty prostate or from some other biological problem, the aforementioned techniques might not work. Masturbation in particular would be difficult for you because you simply would not be able to get erect. For such situations, prostate massage is an excellent option. It can result in intense orgasms and can allow you and your partner to engage in actual sex with each other. There is a step by step process by which you can engage in a prostate massage either on your own or with your partner.

Empty your Bowels

This is a very important part of the process. You would probably at any given time have feces in your rectum. Hence, when you insert your fingers into your anus to massage your prostate, you might end up touching your feces which is certainly not something that you would want to do. If your partner touches your feces it would completely kill the mood, which is understandable. Hence, in order to make the massage fun, it is essential that you empty your bowels before you do anything else.

Take a Shower

Cleanliness is an essential part of prostate massages. Just to be sure that you are absolutely clean, take a shower taking special care to wash that particular part of your body. If you simply don't want to take a shower, you can just wash yourself down there instead. Just take special care to clean yourself out completely. A good idea would be to remove the hair from that area too. No matter how much you clean yourself, hair on your backside is going to be a major turn off for your partner. Remove the potential for disruption in your sex by removing the hair from that area.

Cut Your Nails

If you are planning on giving yourself a prostate massage, it would be a good idea to trim your nails. This is because you might end up cutting or nicking yourself if you penetrate your anus with a finger that has long nails. If your partner is giving you a prostate massage, have her trim her nails. If she does not want to she can try wearing gloves while performing the massage. However, it is highly recommended that she cuts her nails, as a proper massage is done without gloves and is a great deal more pleasurable.

Position Yourself

The best position to get to your prostate is with you on your back. Try tucking your knees into your chest, and placing a cushion under your lower back in order to facilitate easier entry. If this position isn't working for you, try out other positions. You can lie down on your side with a single knee raised (not the one that is one the bed). You can also try getting on all fours and curving your lower back. Every man is different, and finding out which position suits you is an important part of getting a good prostate massage.

Lube Up

One thing that you need to keep in mind is that your anus is not really designed for taking in fingers or other objects, it is designed for expelling things. Hence, in order to ensure that you have an easy time finding your prostate, you need to use lubricant. Just add a few drops to your fingers or your partner's fingers if she is the one doing the prostate massage for you. You can even add lube to your anus if that is more comfortable for you. Once the lube has been applied, you are ready to insert your finger in.

This part is rather tricky because people tend to be a little overexcited while doing this. As a result, they end up thrusting their finger in too roughly and end up causing discomfort. Remember, this is masturbation. You are supposed to enjoy this.

When you put your finger in, do it as gently as possible. Feel your way inside slowly, do not force anything. Your anus will slowly open up to you if you are moving properly. If you take it slow, you will slowly feel any obstructions in your way move aside. The key here is to relax. If you are embarrassed or tense in any way, the muscles in your anus are going to clench. When they clench, it is going to become far more difficult for you to reach your prostate.

The lube should help here. Your anus does not have natural lubricants the way a vagina does, but the lube will compensate for that. If your partner is the one who is penetrating your anus, make sure to communicate with them. Ensure that they know whether you are comfortable or not. Remember that they are not feeling what you are feeling, so the clearer you are about your level of comfort the easier it will be for both of you to enjoy the experience.

You or your partner should slide the finger in until the second knuckle. This is usually how much penetration is required in order to reach the prostate, however, the exact location differs from person to person. Try out different areas and angles, tell your partner to feel around inside you for the right spot.

Once he or she hits the spot, you are going to feel a rather different sensation. Apart from the feeling of them being inside you, you are going to start feeling a light buzzing sensation and are going to be filled with an overpowering urge to contract the muscles of your anus. This is natural, and is similar to the response that women have when you touch their G spot.

However, if you clench your muscles your anus might end up pushing your partner's finger out with the exact same peristalsis it uses to push feces out. If your partner tries to fight against the peristalsis, they might end up injuring you slightly. Hence, it is better that you try your best to avoid clenching the muscles when they hit the prostate.

This will take some practice to do because the sensation when they touch the prostate is going to be intense. The first few times you are inevitably going to push your partner's finger out. Eventually, though, when you get used to the sensation you are going to be better able to avoid the clenching of your muscles. This is why it is recommended that you try to practice on yourself before engaging in this activity with a partner. Once you have discovered your own sexual preferences during this activity, it will become easier for you to guide your partner. Knowledge of one's own body is always supposed to come first.

The finger going in should be doing so with the palm facing up. This is because in order to actually reach the prostate, the finger will have to curl upwards. Once you or your partner's finger is inside, have them curl it upwards and you will feel it brushing against your prostate. If you have practiced keeping your muscles loose, your partner will be able to stimulate your prostate quite frequently.

The sensation will increase to the point where you will begin to feel the pleasure spread across your backside. This blooming of pleasure will spread upwards to your lower back and down the back of your thighs. Unlike with regular masturbation, your groin or penis is the last place the pleasure will reach. It is hard to really know when you have achieved orgasm via your prostate. The climax does not arrive suddenly as with real masturbation, but this process does leave you satisfied. It is thus a rather useful substitute for masturbation and can be a great way for you and your partner to have sex in spite of your erectile dysfunction.

Use Sex Toys

You already know how you can use vibrators and butt plugs in order to stimulate your prostate. Prostate stimulation is also a great way to have sex in a same sex relationship. If your partner penetrates your anus, he can stimulate your prostate gland with his penis. This is standard sex practice among homosexual males, but a lot of people don't know that even the receiving partner, or "bottom", can receive sexual pleasure during sex. Hence, erectile dysfunction can prove to be an easily solvable problem if you are gay.

This same basic principle can translate over to heterosexual relationships too. There is a sex toy called a "strap on" which is essentially a belt of sorts on which a dildo is attached. This can allow your female partner to penetrate you and stimulate your prostate gland. This is a perfectly legitimate way to have sex and can allow you and your partner to have sex in an intimate manner. It can also really turn the tables in your sex life, as you would be the receiving partner for a change! You can also use strap ons yourself. If you suffer from erectile dysfunction, your main problem is that you cannot have penetrative sex with your partner. As a result, you might feel that you are not able to achieve the same level of intimacy that other people might have.

By using a strap on you can solve this problem. In both heterosexual and homosexual relationships, if you are suffering from erectile dysfunction you can easily have penetrative sex using a strap on. It removes the need to get an erection entirely, and can allow you to be deeply intimate with your partner. It is important to remember here that the accumulated stress of being unable to satisfy your partner for a long period of time can be an enormous contributing factor in erectile dysfunction. This is an area where using a strap on can help you immensely. By using a strap on, you can alleviate some of the sexual frustration that might have built up within your partner due to the fact that you are unable to get an erection.

Since your partner will be satisfied with you, sexually speaking, you will be under less pressure during sex. You might be able to get an erection without even realizing it!

In this way, using a strap on can be an important stepping stone to penetrative sex with your penis. It can even be considered the final stepping stone. After sexting, phone sex, video sex, mutual masturbation and the use of toys, you can start having sex that is very close to actual penetrative sex using this technique. You will then just be a baby step away from overcoming your erectile dysfunction. You can even change things up in bed. You can use a butt plug on yourself while penetrating your partner with a strap on. You can use a vibrating butt plug that will stimulate your prostate so that you get pleasure during sex as well. You can put anal beads in and have your partner pull them out when she is climaxing so that you can feel pleasure with her.

The possibilities are endless with sex. Just because you have erectile dysfunction doesn't mean that your life has ended. A normal relationship may be impossible, but in today's modern day and age normal no longer exists. With so many options, you may not have a sex life that you can classify as "normal", but you will certainly have one that is fulfilling and enjoyable for both and your partner.

Bear in mind that if the reason for you erectile dysfunction is low blood supply or excess fat, using a strap on will not help you get erect. This would only work if the stress of an unsatisfied partner is keeping you from getting erect. However, using a strap on will alow you to penetrate your partner with an artificial penis, and thrust in the exact same motion that you would if you were using your penis. Hence, in such situations strap ons may be slightly less useful, but they would still be incredibly useful nonetheless.

POWERFUL Treatments for Erectile Dysfunction

You already know that you can tackle erectile dysfunction through lifestyle changes. However, if you have been suffering from the sexual dysfunction for a long period of time, you probably don't have patience for such long term treatments. Doctors can provide a number of treatments that are medical in nature. If you are looking for such a treatment just go to your doctor and talk about it. The most commonly prescribed pill is viagra, and there are several others that are just as effective.

However, the problem with such medicines is that they tend to have side effects attached to their use. Using Viagra is never just using Viagra. Apart from increased blood flow to your penis, you will also suffer dizziness, potential nausea and other side effects. This does not mean that medical treatments for erectile dysfunction are in any way bad for you. They are the best way to get your dysfunction out of your life. However, reading about medicines in a book is going to be of no help to you, because you have a doctor who is more than willing to prescribe some for you.

Still, it is important to get to know the various options you have. This book will describe your various medical options along with the following:

Natural Treatments

A lot of medicines use natural ingredients in them. The Earth is rich with nutrients and chemicals that have been created for the sole purpose of helping humans with problems such as erectile dysfunction. When the chemicals are extracted, a lot of the residual trace materials are left behind. Hence, natural treatments that go to the root of medicine are quite effective because they have not been processed or sterilized. This is going to be the first section of this particular chapter.

Exercises

There are a number of exercises that you can do which would end up helping you get erect once more. These include exercises designed to target the muscles that are specifically within the same area as your penis, as well as general exercises that you can include in your fitness routine that are quite good at redirecting blood flow to your groin and alleviating erectile dysfunction. Additionally, this section of the book is going to advise you on how frequently to do exercises as well as how you can incorporate them into your daily routine.

Mechanical Solutions

Medicines and exercises aren't the only way that we can get over erectile dysfunction. There are a number of machines and gadgets that actually redirect blood to your penis without you having to worry about lifestyle changes or exercises. As far as immediate solutions go, you cannot get any better than a mechanical solution. The various gadgets that are good for erectile dysfunction are mentioned in this section of the book, as are the various contraindications against these gadgets so that you can make an informed decision about whether you are going to use them or not.

Medicines, Medical Practitioners and Medical Therapies

Viagra

Viagra pills are a godsend for anyone who is suffering from erectile dysfunction. This medicine, along with other similar medicines such as Cialis and Levitra, are made of phosphodiesterase-5 inhibitors. These inhibitors affect your body in such a way that you end up getting a lot more blood flow to your penis. This makes it a lot easier for you to get an erection, as it solves one of the most important problems that might be causing you to have a difficult time getting an erection: a lack of blood flow.

Like all medicines, these drugs have side effects. These side effects include headaches as well as congestion, essentially a blocked nose. It is important that you ask your doctor before taking these pills, because there are certain instances where Viagra or similar drugs cannot be used if you are already taking certain other drugs. For example, if you are taking nitroglycerine, taking Viagra can result in low blood pressure. In some instances, low blood pressure caused by ingesting Viagra while regularly taking nitroglycerine has even resulted in death. Stay safe and ask your doctor before taking any of these drugs.

Penile Injections

This treatment seems rather radical to some, but if you are among the twenty percent of men for whom viagra does not do a thing, or if you simply cannot take oral medication, the penile injections is an excellent option. The results are instantaneous. If you want to have sex, just give yourself a penile injection and you will be erect in no time. However, there are some major side effects to using this treatment.

The first side effect is not all that serious. It is essentially a burning sensation inside your penis. This might be just the medicine working its magic, but on the off chance that it is an allergic reaction it is important that you call your doctor if this ever happens. The other side effect is priapism, which is an erection that lasts more than four hours. It is painful, and you will have to see a doctor in order to make it go down. However, it is important that you bear in mind that penile injections are effective for five out of every six men that try it. With odds like that, it's worth giving it a shot for instant relief.

MUSE is for people who are either unable to get results from get from Viagra or do not want to take pills, and at the same time do not want penile injections either. This is understandable. After all, sticking a needle in your penis every time you need to have sex is not exactly the most attractive thing one can do, and just thinking about that level of discomfort can put a lot men off having sex permanently.

MUSE stands for medicated urethral system for erection. It is basically a pill that can be inserted via a device that you get with the pill into your penis. The device slides into the opening of your penis and deposits the pills there, where it dissolves. The benefit is that you do not need to inject your penis, but for a lot of people inserting something into their urethra isn't exactly a pleasurable idea either. The problem with MUSE is that using it can result in some pretty serious side effects. These side effects include a burning sensation, aching in your penis, a reddish hue after you have injected the pill and in some extreme cases minor bleeding can occur.

Implants

Women aren't the only ones who can get implants. If you suffer from erectile dysfunction, you can get implants as well to solve your problem. There are two different implants that you can get in order to get over your erectile dysfunction. The first of these is essentially a cylinder that is placed inside your penis. Along with this cylinder, you will be given a pump as well as fluid. If you want to have intercourse, you can just manually pump the fluid into the cylinder and make your penis erect so that you can have sex.

The other surgical option is the implanting of a long, malleable road similar to a gooseneck lamp that can be used to put your penis into position whenever you want to have sex. This is similar to a prosthesis, and is permanent. It can be removed once but once it was been removed putting it back in becomes impossible. The problem here is that both of these procedures are incredibly invasive. They involve long processes whereby actual objects are placed inside your penis. Your penis might get irreversibly damaged in the process of putting these implants in, and the long term effect of having such implants could be that your penis might get malformed and stretched out of shape.

Additionally, these implants are life altering. You will no longer be able to urinate properly, as your penis is never going to be flaccid. This is why these implants are usually reserved only for the most extreme cases that come by, where no other alternative solution can be found. The most common situations where these implants are used is when the victim of a car crash or some other form of accident ends up suffering an injury to his spinal cord. As a result, he becomes paralyzed from the waist down and there is no solution that would allow him to have a natural erection anymore.

Such extreme solutions are not recommended for people who suffer from ordinary erectile dysfunction, and in most cases doctors simply won't perform the surgery on you unless you absolutely need it. It is better that you use the previous options that were given as alternatives to penetrative sex, as they will allow you to have a normal sex life without requiring you to undergo an invasive and dangerous procedure that could result in irreparable damage to your body.

Therapy

Couples therapy is one area where people tend to shy away from if it concerns matters of sex. However, there is a special form of therapy, called sex therapy, which you can use in order to get past your erectile dysfunction. This is useful mostly in situations where the erectile dysfunction is caused by mental blockages. Stress, anxiety, shame, all of these things are perfectly legitimate factors that can affect your sex life. Hence, if you are suffering from erectile dysfunction and cannot find anything wrong with your prostate, and indeed nothing else with your body is wrong, then sex therapy may be your best option.

When you attend sex therapy, you are going to discover something very important: one of the most important factors affecting you is the fight or flight response. This is an ancient facet of human psychology that stretches all the way back to when we were still prey, and there were predators out there that could chase us. When we would be in dangerous situation where our life was in peril, our body would fill us with adrenaline so that we may either fight the entity that is posing a danger to us or flee. In a fight or flight response, you would need your blood flow redirected to your brain, so that you can judge the situation and see what kind of response is best, your arms, so that you can fight the thing that is posing a danger to you if the need arises, and your legs so that you can run as fast as you can.

Since blood flow is being redirected to so many different parts of your body, there is none left for your penis. No one needs an erection when they are fighting a foe, or so the body thinks.The problem in the modern day and age that we live in is that we experience the same old fight or flight responses in much more mundane situations. An example of this would be when you are about to have sex. If you are inexperienced with sex or are, for whatever reason, self conscious about the way you look, your body would feel the same rush it would have felt ten thousand years ago if it was faced with a predator.

As a result, a lot of the blood flow is redirected from your groin and taken to your arms and legs, as well as your brain. Since there is no blood flow, you will be unable to get an erection. By going to sex therapy you are going to be able to understand this very important fact about erectile dysfunction. You can also use sex therapy to ascertain what your emotional state is. A lot of the time, your erectile dysfunction might be caused by you being depressed. It is very possible to be depressed without knowing it, but going to sex therapy will allow you to rationalize the way you feel, facilitating a much more stable emotional state. Another area where sex therapy can help you is performance anxiety. The majority of the time, performance anxiety is needless. It is based on unrealistic expectations instilled in you by pornography. A significant minority is caused by genuine concerns such as premature ejaculation, which would end up causing you to get so stressed that you would no longer be able to get an erection. Both of these situations can be helped significantly by going to sex therapy. You can talk out your fears with your counselor and get over them, thereby allowing you to get over your erectile dysfunction.

Hormone Therapy

One of the causes of erectile dysfunction is a low amount of testosterone in the body. This is usually coupled with low libido as well, and can be addressed by using hormone therapy. Hormone therapy essentially involves injecting yourself with testosterone. You can also use gels and patches that you will place upon your skin, through which the testosterone will be absorbed into the blood stream.

Once you begin taking testosterone, you are going to start feeling an increased desire for sex. This will at least make you passionate enough to use some of the alternate techniques that have been discussed in the previous chapter. One problem here is that testosterone does not improve blood flow to the penis. If you are suffering from that particular type of erectile dysfunction, testosterone won't be able to help you.

Additionally, taking testosterone can result in some serious side effects. Acne is a guaranteed side effect of taking testosterone, but some more major side effects can include an unnatural growth of your breasts as well as enlargement of your prostate. Only take testosterone if it has been prescribed by a doctor. There are situations where taking it could result in adverse health effects, such as if you suffer from prostate problems.

Shockwave Therapy

This is a rather extreme way that you can treat your erectile dysfunction. By using electroshock therapy, or shockwave therapy, you are going to essentially rearrange the away your body makes flood flow within it. It is a reprogramming of your blood vessels in a way, and can stimulate major blood flow to your penis in particular. This is because it facilitates a process called revascularization. Through this process, your body can re grow or repair damaged blood vessels.

When this happens, blood flow is promoted and your body becomes better able to transport blood to that particular area.

This has only been used so far to treat people who are recovering from heart attacks. It has been used only in very controlled situations for people who were suffering extreme cases of erectile dysfunction. Hence, no side effects are known yet. This is still a very new therapy, and has not been made available to the public. However, within a few years shockwave therapy may just become the single best way for you to overcome your erectile dysfunction, and it is important that you know as much about it as you can before it comes to the open market.

Natural Treatments

Ginseng

Ginseng is widely regarded as an excellent remedy for a variety of different ailments. It has been used in treating arthritis and has even started being included in a number of energy drinks. Ginseng is also widely known for being an excellent cure for erectile dysfunction, particularly red ginseng. Taking about a couple grams of red ginseng a day has positive results in abut seventy five percent of men, and considering that it helps tackle a number of other issues and has negligible side effects is certainly a bonus.

Golden Root

Golden root, also known as Rhodiola Rosea, is another natural remedy that has been scientifically proven to help alleviate erectile dysfunction. In a clinical trial conducted by a team of scientists, it was ascertained that taking about one hundred and fifty milligrams of golden root a day has about the same effect as ginseng. The bonus with golden root is that it vastly improves libido as well as blood flow through the penis. However, golden root is not as readily available as ginseng which means that your choice between either roots will inevitably result in a give and take.

DHEA

The adrenal gland is responsible for producing adrenaline, but it is also responsible for producing DHEA. This is a secondary hormone that your body can actually convert into testosterone, which makes it a great way to improve libido and make yourself more physically able to have sex. There is a dietary supplement that is composed of yam and soy that you can consume. It is scientifically proven that almost half of the cases of erectile dysfunction are related, more or less, to low levels of DHEA in the body. Hence, consuming a DHEA supplement is a great bet at helping your erectile dysfunction.

L-Arginine

Low amino acid levels are an important factor in erectile dysfunction. One amino acid in particular is known to be important to alleviating erectile dysfunction: L-Arginine. This amino acid is primarily responsible for the production of nitric oxide in the body. The primary function of nitric oxide is to help dilate blood vessels. The constriction of blood vessels is one of the primary causes of erectile dysfunction. Hence, by consuming supplements with LArginine in them, your body will end up producing more nitric oxide which will allow more blood to flow to your penis, thereby taking care of your erectile dysfunction.

Acupuncture

Acupunture has long been known to be an excellent source of relief for a number of things. This includes erectile dysfunction. In fact, several ancient texts have been discovered that have shown that acupuncture has been used for years to treat such conditions. Acupuncture works by altering the energy meridians that are present in all of use. By applying acupuncture techniques, you will be able to regulate the flow of energy in your body and facilitate a more healthy overall system. One of the aspects that this affects is blood flow. According to ancient Chinese philosophy, erectile dysfunction is caused by the energy nexuses that are present within your penis getting clogged. This is inevitable, because a lot of energy goes through these nexuses every day. A clog is inevitable, but this does not mean that it cannot be fixed.

By applying acupuncture techniques, you will be able to smoothen out the flow of energy to your penis. By piercing the points that pertain to the energy nexuses connected to your groin, a professional acupuncture therapist will be able to solve your erectile dysfunction problem as long as it is not caused by any biological or mechanical factors. Acupuncture has a spotty history, but overall, if one looks at the various clinical trials that have been conducted, one would see that about half the people that engage in acupuncture therapy are able to enjoy a much more fulfilling sex life. About forty percent of people who undergo acupuncture therapy have reported being able to get erect with much more ease then they were able to before. Additionally, a quarter of the men who underwent acupuncture therapy reported never suffering from erectile dysfunction again.

It may seem like pseudoscience, but acupuncture therapy has been known to be effective at least some of the time, and that is more than a lot of medicines can say. If nothing else has worked, give acupuncture therapy a try. It's worked for thousands of people before, it might just end up working for you.

Pycnogenol

Much like L-Arginine, pycnogenol can help your body to create nitric oxide. This can be very useful, as it will allow your body to more easily transport blood through your blood vessels. Pycnogenol is a plant product that is derived from tree bark. It is truly a miracle drug, that is often combined with other natural remedies, such as L-Arginine, to create a total remedy for erectile dysfunction. As far as natural remedies go, pycnogenol is possible the single most effective way to get over your erectile dysfunction. When combined with L-Arginine, pycnogenol is even more effective than a number of accepted medicines such as Viagra.

In a clinical trial conducted where participants took the combination of the two natural remedies, four out of every five participants was able to engage in full penetrative sex only two months after taking the combination regularly. As for the remaining twenty percent, most of them were able to regain full sexual ability after a further month of taking this combination of natural remedies. This brought the success rate of this treatment up to an astounding 92%. In the end, only two out of every twenty five participants reported seeing no improvement after taking the drug.

If one takes into consideration the possibility that at least have of these people were taking the treatment incorrectly, this means that the drug has almost a hundred percent success rate. This is far higher than any other drug on the market, which makes this treatment truly worth looking into.

Exercises

Push Ups

Since kegels have already been covered, and by now you have probably tried them six ways to Sunday, it is time for you to learn about other exercises that can help alleviate your erectile dysfunction.

When you think of the pushup you may not think that it is a particularly effective treatment for erectile dysfunction. After all, it is meant to exercise your upper body, such as your chest and shoulder muscles. How can pushups possibly help your erectile dysfunction, which has to do with a part of your body that is far removed from your upper body?

The first major way in which it helps is by improving blood circulation in your body. If you are suffering from poor circulation, it is important that you exercise in order to get your body into the practice of pumping blood to its various areas more efficiently.

Apart from this, pushups help greatly by strengthening your core. This includes the muscles of your abdomen as well as your lower back and, the most important muscles of all, your pelvic muscles. In order to stabilize yourself during pushups, you are going to have to strengthen your core muscles, which in turn means that your pelvic muscles are strengthened. This makes it a lot easier for you to get an erection, firstly because your pelvic muscles will become more powerful, and secondly because exercising your pelvic muscles is going to encourage blood flow to that particular part of your body. More blood flow means that it will be easier for you to get an erection.

Try to do about twenty to thirty pushups a day. You don't need to push yourself, just do enough that you get your blood pumping. Just remember to do them at least three and at most six time a week for the best results.

The Plank

The plank is vastly different from the pushup, but it just as important at helping you overcome your erectile dysfunction. The plank essentially involves you face down, resting your upper body with your elbows and toes.

The way to do this is to get into position as if you were about to do a pushup and then descend until the length of your lower arm is what you are balancing your upper body with. Maintain this position for about a minute and then start doing pushups. You can use this as an interim between pushups in order to make your breather more intense. The more exercise you fill into a small space of time, the more effective your workout is going to be.

The benefit of the plank is that it targets your core just like pushups do. The difference is that with the plank you put a lot more focus on your groin and pelvic muscles. By mixing the plank up with pushups you are going to get your blood flowing and will then be essentially directing it to your pelvis which is going to make this workout super effective at alleviating your erectile dysfunction.

Trampoline

A trampoline is tons of fun. It is a great way to bond with your kids, it's exhilarating, and it helps you slough off the stress of a long day and enjoy yourself. It also helps a great deal with erectile dysfunction. This is because trampoline jumping directs blood entirely to your lower body. One rather interesting fact about trampoline jumping is that the muscle that is used most while engaging in this activity is actually the pelvic muscle.

This makes trampoline jumping rather unique. It is one of the only exercises, apart from kegels, that puts emphasis on the pelvic muscles. An additional benefit of trampoline jumping is that it gets your blood flowing. While you are engaging in this activity, you are going to have a high pulse which means your blood is going to be flowing fast. Since the muscle that you are using the most right now is in your pelvis, a lot of this blood is going to end up flowing to your groin.

This influx of blood is going to end up making it a lot easier for you to get an erection later on when you are trying to have sex.

Gadgets

Electrostimulation Devices

These devices are a great solution for men who do not want to take any kind of medical treatment for their erectile dysfunction. The great benefit of this solution is that it involves no major medication, and is in general just a more intense form of prostate massage. These devices look like little pencils with wider ends that are made of metal. All you really have to do is insert it into your anus and turn it on, after which an electric charge will begin to course through it and stimulate your prostate.

This is an excellent way to promote the health of your prostate gland. If you are looking to increase the amount of testosterone in your body, or if you want to experience more pleasurable orgasms by stimulating your prostate, you can use these devices to help you get the job done.

Electrostimulation is an incredibly effective way to solve the problem of erectile dysfunction. Since your prostate is getting so heavily stimulated, within a week or so of regular use you are going to have so much blood flowing there that you will be able to get incredible erections without much effort, decidedly solving your problem of erectile dysfunction. Electrostimulation is not the sole realm of these wands, however. There are rings that you can place around your cock that will get the job done as well. These rings send a mild current through your penis that will get you hard in a surprisingly short amount of time. As it turns out, electricity on your penis ends up promoting a great deal of blood flow.

You can also get electrolytic creams that will make it a lot easier for you to conduct electricity through your penis, as well as prevent the chance of getting rashes with having the ring on for so long. You can try using a combination of these two electrostimulation devices. Both of these devices being used concurrently is an excellent way to ensure a healthy supply of testosterone and a large and continuous blood supply to that part of your body.

Cock Rings and Vacuum Pumps

By using a pump, you can create a vacuum of blood in your penis. This will result in a great deal of blood rushing back into your penis, thereby engorging the spongy tissue and making your penis rigid and erect. The problem here is that the blood invariably goes rushing back down into your body. In order to stop this, you can use a cock ring. Cock rings cut off blood supply to your penis, thereby making it impossible for your body to suck the blood that has rushed into it back out.

The only problem here is that the cock ring can only be used for about twenty minutes before it can start causing damage to your blood vessels in that part of your body. Hence, cock rings and vacuum pumps are a short term solution that is to be used only when you are about to have sex.

Confidence & Misconceptions

You probably already know that one of the most sever causes of erectile dysfunction is actually a lack of confidence. Since this is such an important issue, you probably already know that there are several different options that you can try out in order to fix it. A lot of these options are going to be discussed in this chapter. The first of these options is, of course, counseling. The majority of erectile dysfunction cases are caused by performance anxiety or other such issues, and the best way to overcome these issues is to go to sex therapy or attend counseling sessions. There are several benefits to this, and a lot of tips that you can use, all of which will be discussed in this chapter.

Apart from these therapies, you are also going to be taught about common misconceptions surrounding erectile dysfunction. These misconceptions often end up causing more stress, which ends up resulting in an increased risk of erectile dysfunction. Finally, you will be given some tips about how to build up confidence and make it easier for yourself to get outside of your head in the bedroom. Remember, chances are that the only person that is stopping you from having enjoyable sex is you, so follow these tips provided in this chapter and be amazed as your erection comes back to you.

Sex Therapy

There are a number of things that you should know about sex therapy. Knowing these things is important because they will help you to get into a position where you will be able to get the most out of your sex therapy. Some of these things would even help assuage any doubts you might be having about attending sex therapy. Here is a list of things that you should know about sex therapy before you begin:

Sex Therapy is For Everyone

One of the major reasons that some people are hesitant to attend sex therapy is that they thing it is meant for people who are sexually deviant in some way. The general opinion about sex therapy in society is that it is reserved for pedophiles or people with uncontrollable and unnatural fetishes. This is not the case at all.

Sex therapy is a normal form of counseling. People go there because of abnormal sexual preferences, they go there in order to discuss body image issues, and they also go there in order to get over the stress that is causing them to suffer from erectile dysfunction.

By attending sex therapy, you are not going to be any different from anyone else. The people who would be sitting with you in the waiting room are probably not rapists, and you are most certainly not going to be judged for going there. In fact, doing so is a positive move, one that shows that you are willing to work on your problems.

You're Going to Learn about your Sexual Psychology

The primary think that you and your counselor are going to be discussing is going to have nothing to do with your fetishes, it is going to have to do with how you perceive yourself. This is an extremely important part of suffering from erectile dysfunction, and you can be sure that your counselor is going to want to discuss it. Whenever your fetishes or preferences come up, it is just going to be part of the process of learning how you perceive sex. This is not someone you donâ€™t know sitting in front of you. The person you are speaking to is a sex professional, they have been taught to look into your perceptions and discover the source of your anxiety.

You are going to learn a thing or two that you might not like. This is another normal part of sex therapy. Nobody would like having to hear about things that make them anxious, no matter how much they are told that it is going to help them. Hence, when you are talking to your sex therapist, it is important that you discuss how you are feeling about what is being discussed.

Just try your best not to get offended. Whatever the sex therapist is telling you is entirely confidential, and a good sex therapist is never going to judge you for what you share with them. If you feel judged or embarrassed by the way your sex therapist is treating you, get yourself a new one immediately. Feel free to comment on what your sex therapist is revealing about your psychology. Sometimes sex therapists intentionally say things to see how you will react, and based on your reaction they will able to glean more information about the root of your problem.

You Will Get Practice Suggestions

One of the most important aspects of a therapists job is to suggest ways in which you can improve your sex life. A lot of people get embarrassed by this because sex has been such a taboo topic for so long. Think of your sex therapist as your doctor. Whatever your doctor says, any comments that he or she makes, is going to be done in a professional capacity. The exact same goes for your sex therapist. It is important that you are open about your preferences when this stage of therapy emerges. If your therapist does not know what sort of things you like in bed, her or she would not be able to suggest adequate sex exercises for you to do.

When you are given homework to do, don't be shy about doing it. And whatever the results are, just remember that there is no wrong way to do something. With these suggestions, your sex therapist is going to be forming a profile of your sexual psyche. Whatever you can't do is not mandatory until your therapist actually says so. By following your therapist's suggestions, you will be able to get over your erectile dysfunction quite quickly.

Take Your Partner Along

You may be embarrassed to do so, but taking your partner along is an important part of the process. Nobody wants to be laid bare this way in front of someone they love, but sometimes it is the only way to truly get past what you are feeling. If you are unwilling to let your partner in or discuss such things with them, just keep in mind that your partner is suffering just as much as you are. Being unable to engage in a normal sexual relationship can have an effect on anybody.

Hence, by bringing your partner in to therapy with you, you are going to be able to make a lot more headway. Firstly, your partner will be able to discuss his or her sexual preferences as well. As a result, your therapist will be able to prescribe more accurate activities and exercises for the two of your to do. Additionally, your partner can also discuss any concerns he or she might have about your sex life. It is important that the two of you get through this ordeal together, and the best way to do this is to go to sex therapy sessions together.

A lot of people suffer from the misconception that if they go to sex therapy they will have to take their clothes off. This is because we associate sex with nudity, so naturally when we think of a sex therapist the image that comes to mind is someone that would hover over your naked body, dictating how you masturbated and telling you what you were doing wrong.

This is actually the exact opposite of what a sex therapist should do. You will never be asked to get naked, nor will you ever be touched in an inappropriate way. However, there are a lot of situations where a sex therapist would use their position of power to get someone naked in their office. This is just another way that perverts and deviants sexually assault people. If you are ever asked to take your clothes off while engaging in sex therapy, just remember that you are not required to do so, and that this is definitely not part of any true form of sex therapy. The best thing to do in such a situation would be to leave immediately and change your sex therapist.

Be Careful While Choosing a Sex Therapist

If there is one thing you shouldn't be hasty about, it's choosing a sex therapist. You have probably already ascertained from the previous point that there are a lot of sex therapists out there who would use their power to get people to have sex with them. Sex therapy is a rather new profession, and there are still a lot of bugs to get out. This profession tends to attract some people who are just looking for a power dynamic to exploit.

It is thus extremely important that you vet your sex therapist careful before settling on one. Ask for credentials at every turn, and never be afraid to question a therapist's methods. Remember, you are the one who is paying them. They are providing a service to you. You have every right to be upset with how they are doing things. Within reason, try to question your therapist's suggestions. Are the things they are suggesting odd? Do they make you uncomfortable? If this is the case, get a second opinion, and confront your therapist. Just try not to be too hostile, chances are they were just trying to help you.

Sex Therapy is not a Surefire Solution to Erectile Dysfunction

One of the most dangerous misconceptions about sex therapy is that attending sessions will inevitably lead to you recovering from your erectile dysfunction. While sex therapy is an incredibly useful way to overcome he anxieties that might be resulting in your sexual dysfunction, sex therapy is by no means guaranteed to get you out of the woods. It will certainly help, but sometimes your problems are too deep rooted for therapy to fix. Don't get your hopes too high up because disappointment is that last thing you are going to be needing right now.

Additionally, sex therapy will not help if you are suffering from erectile dysfunction as a result of physical problems. Inadequate blood flow, low testosterone levels and all other deficiencies in your body which would have resulted in your erectile dysfunction can never be solved through therapy. However, going to therapy might benefit you by giving you these problems as options. If you need help ascertaining why you are suffering from erectile dysfunction, sex therapy can almost certainly help you there. Just don't expect going to sessions to be the only way you can get cured for sure.

Common Misconceptions about Erectile Dysfunction

Wearing Tight Underwear Causes Erectile Dysfunction

This is a common myth that you frequently hear about. However, it is completely untrue. It is a misconception that is based off of another unrelated medical fact. This fact is that wearing tight underwear keeps testicles too close to the body, which results in higher heat levels than is optimal for sperm production. This results in infertility. However, this infertility and erectile dysfunction are two completely different things. If you suffer from erectile dysfunction, it is unlikely that your sperm count has been affected by this. Additionally, if you are suffering from infertility, than you probably won't have any difficulties getting erect because infertility has nothing to do with the amount of blood that flows into your groin. Thus, wearing tight underwear will not cause erectile dysfunction.

Erectile Dysfunction Means You Don't Like Your Partner

A common source of stress for men with erectile dysfunction is that their inability to get erect means that they do not love their wives, girlfriends or partners. This ends up causing more stress which further exacerbates the erectile dysfunction.

However, there is absolutely no reason to think this way about your partner. Your erectile dysfunction is the result of low blood flow to your penis or a low amount of testosterone in your bloodstream. It has nothing to do with how attractive your partner is, or how much you love him or her. Worrying about something like this will only make your erectile dysfunction worse, so it is better to avoid the topic altogether. If you really feel as if this is the case, talk to your therapist about it. They will be able to at least talk you through the emotions that you are feeling.

Erectile Dysfunction becomes Naturally Inevitable with Age

A common fear that a lot of men have is that when they get old, they are going to end up suffering from erectile dysfunction. This is because there is a tendency among older men to get this sexual dysfunction.

As a result, men who cross their mid forties start to stress out about whether they are going to start suffering from this dysfunction or not. Ironically, this stress ends up causing erectile dysfunction, which further proves the misconception that as you get older you will definitely get erectile dysfunction. Erectile dysfunction is similar to arthritis or cancer. These things are not inevitable as you grow older, they just become more likely. As long as you lead a healthy lifestyle and get adequate amounts of exercise, you are never going to have to worry about erectile dysfunction.

Erectile Dysfunction is Abnormal among Young People

Another common cause of stress for men erectile dysfunction only happens to older men. Getting it while you are young is a sign that you are not sexually virile, or are just deficient in some way.

On the contrary, erectile dysfunction is common among men of every age. If you are leading an unhealthy lifestyle, chances are you are going to end up suffering from erectile dysfunction. It is not a sign that you are somehow sexually inferior, you just need to change some of your habits and you will be absolutely fine. As has been mentioned before, erectile dysfunction is definitely more prevalent among older men. However, just because it is somewhat uncommon among younger men does not mean that you are any less of a man for having it. Don't stress yourself out over it, just take it as natural part of life and get the therapy you need.

The Best Way to Treat Erectile Dysfunction is by Using Medicine

Most people tend to think that if they suffer erectile dysfunction popping a Viagra is the best way to ensure that you don't have to deal with erectile dysfunction any longer. While medicines are effective at assuaging the symptoms of erectile dysfunction, they aren't even the first things doctors recommend in order to get over erectile dysfunction. The first step to getting over erectile dysfunction is altering your lifestyle, taking exercise and following a better diet. If you apply these principles to your life, you will get over your erectile dysfunction without too much struggle.

It is only in more serious cases where doctors start to prescribe medicines, as in such situations it is better to take the medicine and suffer he side effects rather than not take the medicine at all. Hence, medicine is not the best way to combat erectile dysfunctions, diet and exercise is.

Erectile Dysfunction is All in Your Head

While it is true that in most of the cases where erectile dysfunction has become a problem, the main issue lies with anxiety and social stress, it is a misconception that erectile dysfunction can only ever be caused by stress and other such psychological issues. Erectile dysfunction is also caused by a number of physiological problems as well. Low testosterone levels, kidney issues, fat that is blocking blood flow to that part of your body, all of these are legitimate issues that can cause erectile dysfunction.

Hence, if you are suffering from erectile dysfunction, don't automatically assume that it is being caused by your psyche. Doing so might just end up putting more pressure on you when you are unable to get over your sexual dysfunction through therapy and the like.

Erectile Dysfunction Can't be Caused by Riding a Bike

This is one of those rare occasions where a misconception about something not causing erectile dysfunction turns out to be false. Riding a bike is widely considered to be a safe activity that can never cause erectile dysfunction. This is because there are a lot of rumors that go around about erectile dysfunction and none of them appear to be true.

With biking however, the rumor actually is true. By cycling a lot, you put pressure on your groin and restrict blood flow in that area. As a result, the blood vessels get damaged, leading to erectile dysfunction.

How To Build Sexual Confidence

Note Insecurities Down

Whenever you feel insecure about something, just write it down on a piece of paper. When you do this, you are going to make the insecurity something that you can objectively analyze. When you write your insecurity down, read it back to yourself. Question this insecurity, ask yourself why you feel this way. Is the insecurity valid? Is it necessary? Try to find out the source of this insecurity, and ask yourself if that source is even trustworthy.

Eventually you will start to see that a lot of your insecurities are the result of bad perceptions of yourself. You are not actually as bad as you make yourself out to be. However, your perception of yourself remains negative. It is this aspect of your life that you will truly be able to change once you start writing down your insecurities and analyzing them.

Educate Yourself

There is a lot of shame that is commonly attributed to sex. What your preferences are, the way you feel about your body, a lot of these things are judged by people. You are made to feel unusual, a freak as it were. This is why it is so important to start educating yourself about sex. Learn about as many sexual preferences as possible. You will find out that a lot of your preferences are very commonplace. Even the most outlandish ones would be perfectly normal, with legitimate explanations. Unless you are a pedophile, it is highly unlikely that your sexual preferences will be so abhorrent that they would warrant disgust.

The fear of being judged plays a huge role in making men feel stressed out about sex. This stress usually results in erectile dysfunction more often than not.

Do Things That Make you Feel the Way You Want to Feel

We live in exciting times. People no longer have to conform to enforced notions of gender anymore. A man is no longer less of a man if he cries, and he is no longer expected to be burly and stoic. You are, essentially, freer than ever before to be whoever you want to be. This means that a lot of your stress in not valid. Most men feel stressed out because they do not conform to these notions of masculinity. It is a natural occurrence, since this is the first generation that is emerging after those imposed notions of masculinity have been removed.

The best way you can build sexual confidence is being the kind of man you want to be. There are women and men out there with incredibly diverse tastes and preferences. This means that no matter what kind of man you want to be, you can be sure that there will be a host of potential partners for you. Stop worrying about being the "right" kind of man. There is no such thing. By worrying so much about something so meaningless, you are going to end up suffering from erectile dysfunction if you are not suffering from it already.

Have More Sex

The only way you can get confident about sex is by having as much sex as possible. This might seem odd to you, but this really is the best way. If you are stressed out about sex, chances are your erectile dysfunction has not progressed to the point where you are completely unable to get erect. Even if you are, there are so many people in the world who would enjoy the kinkier side to sex that you can be sure that you would find someone willing to acquiesce to your requirements.

By having sex, you will realize that it really isn't that difficult. If you are young, there are plenty of opportunities to have sex. As long as you ensure that you are safe, having sex will help you develop a better body image as well. This is because having sex will instill in you the belief that you are not unattractive. After all, why would anyone have sex with someone unattractive?

Remove the Negatives from your Vocabulary

Being self deprecating is fair, and can be funny in some occasions. However, this is only up to the point where it is amusing and not an actual representation of what you think about yourself. If you are constantly self deprecating, you are going to end up believing some of the things you are saying. Remain positive about your body image, and avoid all negative spaces where people would make you feel bad about yourself.

This is especially important for you as a man who is suffering from erectile dysfunction. If you are in a space where you feel as though you are being ridiculed or made to feel low about your dysfunction, leave that space immediately. The stress that would come from the ridicule will greatly exacerbate your erectile dysfunction.

Look at Real Bodies

Watching porn and looking at male models might leave you with the impression that real men are ripped and muscular, and that they all have large penises. This is not the case at all. Real mean are fat and skinny, they are bald and hairy, and penis size ranges from four all the way to seven inches long. And each and every one of these men has sex. You can too, there is no reason why you are any less than any other man.

In order to form a better body image, try looking at as many real bodies as possible. Try going for amateur porn which would have normal men instead of studio porn where porn stars are chosen for their looks.

Admit the Importance of Body Positivity

For a lot of people, body image issues is something only women suffer from. As a man, you can suffer from them too. Acknowledge this fact. Stressing out over your body image issues is probably what caused your erectile dysfunction in the first place, so try to acknowledge the importance of accepting your body.

Conclusion